The Nature and Nurture of Twins

by

Elizabeth M Bryan MD, MRCP, DCH,

Hon. Consultant Paediatrician and Senior Research Fellow
Queen Charlotte's Maternity and Hammersmith Hospitals, London
Senior Clinical Medical Officer, Hereford Health Authority
President of the Twins Clubs Association

Baillière Tindall · London

Published by BAILLIÈRE TINDALL,
a division of Cassell Ltd,
1 St. Anne's Road, Eastbourne, East Sussex BN21 3UN

First published 1983

ISBN 0 7020 0977 6

Typeset by Scribe Design, Gillingham, Kent
Printed in Great Britain by Nene Litho and bound by Woolnough Bookbinding,
both of Wellingborough, Northants.

British Library Cataloguing in Publication Data

Bryan, Elizabeth M.
  1. Twins   2. Infants—Care and hygiene
  I. Title
  649'.14'4   RJ101

  ISBN 0–7020–0977–6

Contents

Preface

Twins invariably inspire interest and admiration. Each year most of the 7000 British mothers who have twins are told how lucky they are to have them. This is the reaction not only of relatives, neighbours and society in general but also of the medical profession. Few doctors and nurses realize what is involved in looking after and relating to two babies at the same time.

While pursuing a study of placental function in multiple pregnancy in 1974 I had the chance to meet over 100 mothers with their twins. Throughout their first year I saw them regularly, often in their homes. Previously I had known nothing of the problems of having young twins. By the end I had learned a great deal.

Not only had I learned of the immense practical, financial and, not least, the emotional difficulties of looking after two babies but also the paucity of support these mothers received. They had been given little advice. They could find no written information. Many of the paediatricians and family doctors involved had seemed unaware of the problems.

This first impression of needs at once substantial and unmet, has been amply confirmed by many of the 1000 or more parents of twins with whom I have now talked, either in my work as a paediatrician or through the Twins Clubs Association. It is to them I am indebted for most of the examples quoted in the text.

The need for information on twins, and concern about them, has since been demonstrated by the extraordinary response to the founding in 1978 of the Association. In the first 18 months this self-help organization for parents of twins received separate enquiries from over 3000 people including parents of twins, members of the medical profession, teachers and research workers.

This book is primarily for paediatricians but I hope that it will be of interest to anyone concerned with any sort of help to families with twins from conception onwards. Indeed some sections, such as that on schooling, will more directly concern the doctor working in the community than the hospital paediatrician. The book is not a detailed practical guide on the care of twins. Nor is its purpose to give technical details on such aspects as obstetrical procedures or placental examination, for which specialized textbooks are available. Rather it aims to give a comprehensive overview of twinning and of twinship, of the effect of twins on a mother and the rest of the family, on the growth and development of twins from conception to adulthood. It has been written too in the hope that those who read it may gain more insight into what it means to be a mother, father, brother or sister of twins—and not least to be born a twin oneself.

Acknowledgements

In writing on a subject which calls on so many disciplines I have inevitably needed help from a great number and variety of people. Responsibility for the book's contents is of course entirely my own but I must mention some of those to whom I feel particularly indebted. These include Jim Barnes, Barbara Broadbent, Doris Campbell, Averil Clegg, Alison Elliman, Emanuel Lewis, Rosemary Macdonald, Barbara Morgan, Cherry Rowland and Christine Tuck.

I thank Wendy Spicer for her care in typing the manuscript and Ann Saadi, my editor, for her enthusiasm and help.

To Gerald Corney I give special thanks not only for much advice but also for constant support.

Judi Linney and many members of the Twins Clubs Association have given me valuable insights into the pleasures and problems of having twins.

To Ronald Higgins, my husband, my readers may be as grateful as I. Such coherence and fluency as the book offers are the product of his literary skills and without his support I might never have shouldered the task.

The book is dedicated to Pamela Davies in gratitude for her unstinting encouragement and wise counselling over many years.

1. History of Twins

The widespread interest in twins has its own psychological and even philosophical roots. Those cultures—probably most—which believe in the uniqueness of each human life and personality are bemused by the fact that some of us have, or seem to have, an identical copy. This is at once a marvel of nature and some sort of metaphysical insult.

Some would feel that the very possibility of twins not only subtracts from the sense of unique individuality but also creates a kind of existential unease. Many of these feelings are expressed in mythology and in tribal customs associated with twinning.

BIBLICAL TWINS

Twins excited much interest in biblical times. The most famous pair were Esau and Jacob, conceived as a result of Isaac's prayer for his barren wife, Rebekah. Esau and Jacob have been variously described as dizygotic (DZ—see p.16) twins on the grounds of their physical dissimilarity as adults, Esau being a 'hairy man' and Jacob a 'smooth man'. On the other hand, because Esau 'came out red' it has also been suggested that he was an example of the fetofetal transfusion syndrome (see p.46). As the fetofetal transfusion syndrome only occurs in monozygotic (MZ—see p.15) twins the two hypotheses are incompatible.

The idea of conflict between twins, so common in mythology, is exemplified by the struggle that Esau and Jacob were said to have had within the womb for the first birthright. Esau won this round

1

but finally lost when Jacob tricked his father into giving the birthright to him.

Another pair of twins described in Genesis are Pharez and Zarah, the children of Tamai and Judah, who also competed to be delivered first. Zarah presented an arm which was labelled with a red string. Later when the babies were born the string was attached to the second baby showing that Pharez had replaced Zarah in birth order.

MYTHOLOGY

Twins abound in Greek and Roman mythology. Many were either gods themselves or the offspring of gods and as such had supernatural powers. Castor and Pollux, the heroic sons of Zeus and Leda, had powers over the wind and waves and were known as the seafarers' guardians. When Castor was killed in battle Pollux was so desolate that he begged his father to allow him to join his brother. They became the heavenly constellation, Gemini.

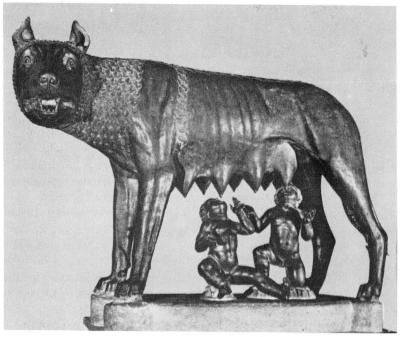

Fig. 1.1. Statue of Romulus and Remus being suckled by the she-wolf. By permission of the Capitoline Museum, Rome.

Romulus and Remus are the most famous twins in Roman mythology. These were the sons of Mars and one of the Vestal Virgins, Sylvia. The babies were to be drowned with their mother in the River Tiber but their cradle reached the bank where they were found and suckled by a she-wolf. There are statues depicting this in both Rome and Siena (Fig. 1.1). When they grew up the two brothers wanted to found a great city but could not agree on a site. In their dispute Romulus killed Remus and then went on to found the city of Rome, over which he ruled for many years.

Narcissus is a much maligned mythological twin. It is sometimes forgotten that he had a twin sister to whom he was devoted. When she died he spent long hours looking at his own reflection in a pool, not out of vanity, but to remind himself of his lost sister.

Motifs of twins are often seen amongst the gods of the Asiatic religions. Sometimes these are depicted as conjoined twins—a figure with two heads or one with several sets of limbs. The Acvin are twin gods in Indian mythology and are believed to look after the weak and oppressed.

In Mexico the ancient Aztecs worshipped the goddess of fertility, Xochiquetzal, whom they believed to be the first mother of twins.

TWINS IN THE ARTS

Writers, poets and artists have all explored the theme of twinship and through their work we can learn much of its various aspects.

Many writers have of course exploited the similarity of twins and the confusion that can spring from it. In his play *Menaechmi* the Roman comic dramatist, Plautus, employed a theme which has since been the basis for countless dramas in many languages. A twin named Menaechmus, who was so like his brother that even their mother could not tell them apart, was lost at the age of seven. Many years later his twin brother, now renamed Menaechmus too, seeks out his lost twin. It is only when strangers start mistaking him for his brother that he realizes that his search will be successful.

Shakespeare sired his own twins, Hamnet and Judith, who were plainly DZ. In his drama, however, he concentrates on the confusion of identity between 'identical' twins. In the *Comedy of Errors* two masters, who appear to be MZ twins, each have one of an MZ pair as their servant. Shakespeare, like many early writers, did not realize that male/female pairs could not be 'identical' twins. In *Twelfth Night* Viola and Sebastian, of whom it was said, 'an

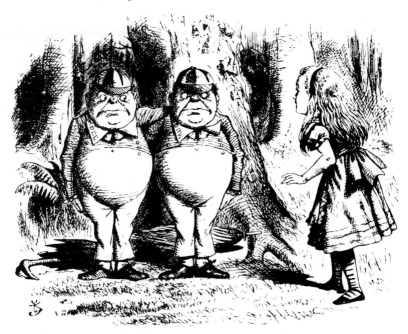

Fig. 1.2. Tweedledum and Tweedledee with Alice. From Lewis Carroll's *Through the Looking Glass and What Alice Found There*. By permission of Macmillan and Co.

apple, cleft in twain is not more twin than these two creatures', enjoyed the confusion they caused.

Tweedledum and Tweedledee in Lewis Carroll's *Through the Looking Glass* must be the most popular pair amongst children (Fig. 1.2).

The immensely close attachment and interdependence of twins are illustrated by Thornton Wilder in *The Bridge of San Luis Rey*. A pair of twins are so close that when one falls in love with a girl there is no space for a third person; this external relationship is so devastating to the twins that it has to be sacrificed. Both twins value their own bond above all. Later Wilder movingly describes the desolation of the survivor after the death of his twin.

CULTURAL AND RELIGIOUS BELIEFS ABOUT TWINS

Throughout history there have been strongly held cultural and religious beliefs about twins in many parts of the world (Gedda 1961; Corney 1975a). Many of these persist today even if usually in modified and less extreme forms. Within the last 20 years an English paediatrician working in Zimbabwe was dismayed to find that one of a pair of premature twins who had been born and successfully nursed in hospital for several months were killed the day after they returned to their own village. It was the custom of the tribe to kill twins.

Attitudes towards twins vary greatly in different parts of the world and even between different tribes within quite small geographical areas. For some twins the difference between being born on one side of the river rather than the other may be that between being welcomed (and even being regarded as having supernatural powers) and being rejected and killed.

Attitudes towards twins have been seen to change over time. Early this century a trader and his family were travelling through the Yoruba territory in Nigeria when his wife was delivered of twins. As he came from a tribe that respected twins the babies were allowed to survive. The trader prospered and it became clear to the Yoruba people that the twins had brought no ill-effect to the family. The Yoruba chiefs therefore decided to change their policy and from then on their own twins were welcomed.

The killing of twins was widespread and has been reported from many parts of Africa and Asia as well as amongst Australian aboriginals and Eskimos. Ideas on the origin of this custom are varied; there are several theories as to why twins were disliked. One is that it is animal-like for a human mother to have more than one baby at a time. Another is that two babies must mean two fathers: the mother must therefore either have committed adultery or have conceived the second baby through an evil spirit. There is often a functional side to the beliefs as well. In a nomadic tribe it is difficult for a mother to carry two babies for many miles and when food is scarce breast-feeding two babies may be impossible. Some tribes killed both babies, some just the second-born or, in mixed-sex pairs, the girl. In some tribes only male/female pairs were killed. They are condemned as it is thought that incest is inevitable either in intrauterine life or later. On the other hand the Bantu positively welcomed male/female pairs as newly weds, and in parts of Japan and the Philippines such pairs were expected to marry.

Aversion to twins was not limited to primitive societies. They were commonly disliked in Japan; in noble families their arrival was kept secret and the second baby might be given to a courtier.

Twins were rejected in parts of South America and this was expressed in the saying 'Papoose double make heap trouble'.

Mothers of twins suffered too. 'May you become the mother of twins' was in some African tribes the strongest curse. Indeed words were unnecessary: two fingers of the right hand pointed towards a woman could have the same terrible effect! In some tribes mothers were killed together with their babies or, if not killed, banished to a distant 'twin town', sometimes for life. When the presence of a second baby was discovered the mother was sometimes moved, still in labour, from the village so that she did not contaminate the area. When the second baby was born unexpectedly, elaborate rituals of purification were performed.

In parts of East Africa the mother was shunned until the babies had cut their first teeth.

On the whole, fathers of twins were let off lightly. Some North American Indians insisted on a period of abstinence from meat and fish, which must have been hard for a hunter. In parts of Peru the father had to abstain from salt, pepper and sexual intercourse for 6 months—an intriguing triad.

Customs Associated with Twins

In some parts of the world there are elaborate ceremonies and rituals associated with twins.

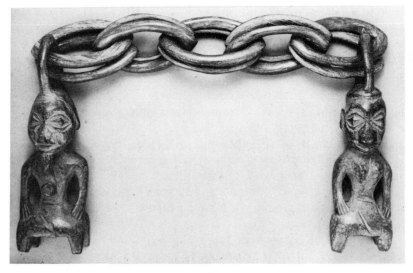

Fig. 1.3. Wooden twin images from West Africa, linked by chain. The whole is made from one piece of wood.

Twin Images

Carved wooden images of twins are common in some parts of Africa particularly in the Ibeji cult of the Yoruba. Ibeji, literally meaning 'to beget two', is used either as a general term for twins or specifically for Orisha, the goddess of twins. Through the traffic of slaves the Ibeji cult has spread to many parts of South America and the Caribbean. Some images are memorials to twins who have died. Often the twin images, sometimes in large numbers, are used for special rituals and kept in places of worship (Fig. 1.3).

Weather

Twins were often believed to have supernatural powers, both good and bad, over the weather. Egyptian twin gods Shu and Tefnut were respectively the wind and rain gods and the powers of Castor and Pollux have already been mentioned.

In parts of eastern and southern Africa twins were thought to cause famine due to drought or flood and were therefore killed immediately to prevent such catastrophes.

Many North American Indians also held twins responsible for the climatic conditions. The Mohaves, for instance, believed that twins came from the sky using lightning, thunder and rain as their means of descent. The Tsimshian, when praying for a storm to abate, would say 'calm down breath of twins'. Many South American tribes attributed aspects of the weather to the mood and behaviour of twins. Indeed twins were used to forecast the weather according to their state of health. When they were feeling well the weather should be clement. When they had a headache or indigestion a storm was likely.

Death of a Twin

It has often and widely been believed that a twin would rarely survive the death of the other and if a twin does survive he is thought likely to be exceptionally strong as the possessor of the vitality of both.

In Sussex it was thought that a single surviving twin had special healing powers, that he or she could cure, for example, thrush by breathing into the mouth of the sufferer.

In some parts of Africa surviving twins may carry a wooden image representing their dead twin around their neck or waist. This gives company to the survivor and a refuge for the spirit of the dead.

Twin Names

Twins in many African tribes are given fixed names. Amongst the Yoruba the firstborn twin is called Taiwo (he who has the first taste of the world) and the second called Kainde or Kehinde (he who lags behind). The younger sibling of twins is called Idowu (the servant of twins) and this name is also given to the third member of triplets. Subsequent children are called Alaba (the servant of Idowu) and Idogbe. In other parts of Africa twins are called Ochin and Omo, Tali and Bali, Buth and Duoth.

The children of twins may also have special names. In one tribe, for example, the firstborn is Dosu (girl, Devi), the second Dosavi (Dohnevi) and the third Donyo (Dosovi).

Conception

For those who wish for twins certain foods are thought to do the trick. In parts of the Far East a double banana, chestnut or millet seed added to the diet of a mother is confidently believed to cause twins. Nearer home, in mediaeval Scotland a tumbler full of water from the well in St. Mungo was supposed to ensure a twin birth.

Some North American Indians say that twins occur if the mother lies on her back instead of on her side during labour, so that the fetus splits into two. Others believe that too much work during pregnancy can result in twins.

Fertility

Twins themselves are thought by some to induce fertility. In Wales they were invited to weddings to ensure children for the newly weds.

Twins are evidence of high fertility in the mother and some tribes believe that this fertility can be transferred to the land. Mothers of twins may be required to join in elaborate rituals in order to ensure a good harvest.

OLD WIVES' TALES

False beliefs about the biology of twins have been rife throughout the centuries. In mid-seventeenth century Europe it was still thought that boy and girl twins could not co-exist in the same uterine cavity because of the '*horror incestus*'. Even today parents may be influenced by superstitions. An elderly midwife recalled how, when one of her patients was delivered of twins, the husband immediately sued for divorce on the grounds of adultery. Two babies must have meant two fathers.

Parents of MZ girls may still sometimes worry about their children's fertility. One mother anxiously sought advice as to which of her 4-year-old girls would be infertile. For 4 years she had lived under the painful misapprehension that only one of her MZ twins would be able to bear children.

Those who have a boy and a girl may be concerned about the fertility of the girl. The farmer father of a boy and girl pair also assumed that his daughter would be infertile as he knew that when a cow gives birth to twins of different sexes the heifer is sterile—the so-called freemartin—due to virilization by hormones from the bull fetus. He did not realize, however, that the pattern of vascular anatomoses in human and bovine placentae is different.

THE STUDY OF TWINS

Scholars and philosophers have always been fascinated by twins. Relatively few scientists have shown the same interest, however. Hippocrates thought about twins and decided that they were conceived by the division of a sperm into two parts and that each part penetrated one of the uterine horns. A number of others including Democritus, Empedocles and Aristotle had ideas on the origin of twins.

Interest in obstetrical aspects was kindled in the Renaissance period and anxiety was expressed over the dangers of exsanguination of the second twin after the firstborn's cord had been cut.

It is perhaps surprising that the value of twins as a research tool was not appreciated until the second half of the nineteenth century. This may have been partly because the distinction between MZ and DZ twins was still not clearly defined. Accurate determination of zygosity has indeed only recently become possible.

Twin research was revolutionized by Sir Francis Galton. It was he who realized that twins could be of value in the study of the effects of heredity and environment on human development. His classic *The History of Twins as a Criterion of the Relative Powers of Nature and Nurture* (1875) is a memorial to his pioneering work.

Before Galton's time twins were regarded as an interesting phenomenon and an obstetrical challenge but of no material or substantial relevance to the rest of the population.

2. The Biology of Twinning

Long before sophisticated methods of determining the zygosity of twins were developed it was recognized that at least two types existed—identical and fraternal. These are otherwise termed monozygotic (MZ), monozygous or uniovular and dizygotic (DZ), dizygous or binovular.

MZ twins arise from the early division of a single fertilized ovum. Evidence for this is provided in at least three ways: by conjoined twins; by the single chorion found in some twin placentae; and from typing of genetic markers. On the other hand, DZ twins occur as the result of fertilization of two separately released ova.

There has been speculation as to the existence of a third type of twin (Mijsberg 1957; Bulmer 1970; Corney and Robson 1975). Such pairs, it is thought, might arise from the division of an ovum whose resulting parts are then fertilized by different spermatozoa. These uniovular dispermatic twins would therefore be intermediate between MZ and DZ. The embryological possibility of this third type is clearly there and after several fruitless lines of investigation the first supportive evidence has been provided by Nance (1981) who describes a twin fetus which was thought to have arisen from the fertilization of a polar body. The twins were thus monovular, but not monozygotic. In this case the fetus was acardiac and thus HLA typing and chromosome analysis were performed. An apparently normal monovular dizygotic twin might well remain unrecognized (Goldgar and Kimberling 1981).

INCIDENCE

Twinning rates vary greatly in different parts of the world (Table 2.1) largely due to variations in DZ twinning. The incidence of MZ twins appears to be relatively, and remarkably, constant all over the world—between 3 and 4 per 1000 maternities.

In both the UK and the USA the incidence of twin deliveries is now about 10 per 1000 (Registrar General 1979), whereas in parts of Nigeria it has been reliably reported to be as high as 45 per 1000 (Nylander 1967, 1970a). In general it appears that the negroid races have the highest incidence, mongoloid races the lowest and Caucasians and Asian Indians, intermediate. Occasionally, as for instance in parts of Finland (Eriksson and Fellman 1973), an isolated community may have an unexpectedly high twinning rate presumably due to inbreeding in a genetically prone population. The DZ twinning rate has been falling over the past decade at least in developed countries and the possible reasons will be discussed later in this chapter.

The incidence of twins in the adult population is always lower than that at birth because both perinatal and infant mortality are higher in twins than singletons (see p.95).

Figures from many developing countries must be interpreted with caution (Nylander 1975a). If the data are obtained from hospital records the incidence of twins may be abnormally high as twin deliveries, together with other high-risk pregnancies, are over-represented amongst hospital deliveries. Conversely, national records may underestimate the number of twins, as babies may not be registered as twins especially in areas where they are unwelcome. Twin taboos are still strong in some African tribes (see Chapter 1).

Sex Ratio

Although there are slightly more male than female twin births, the sex ratio (male: female) is lower than in singletons. In triplets there is actually a preponderance of females (Bulmer 1970; Czeizel and Acsádi 1971) (Table 2.2).

The higher incidence of females amongst multiple compared with single births is not limited to MZ twins. It seems, therefore, that intrauterine influences common to both types of twins must be responsible for the difference. Perhaps the less favourable conditions of a multiple pregnancy raises the mortality rate of the more

Table 2.1. Rates of twinning in different parts of the world. Adapted from Nylander (1975*b*) by permission of the author and W.B. Saunders Co. Ltd.

Author	Date of investigation	Place	Population	Incidence of twins/1000 births			Other information
				Total	DZ	MZ	
Bulmer (1960)		*Europe*					
	1951–53	Spain	National birth statistics	9.1	5.9	3.2	Standardized for maternal age
	1955–56	Portugal	"	10.1	6.5	3.6	
	1946–51	France	"	10.8	7.1	3.7	
	1950	Belgium	"	10.9	7.3	3.6	
	1952–56	Austria	"	10.9	7.5	3.4	
	1901–53	Luxembourg	"	11.4	7.9	3.5	
	1950–55	West Germany	"	11.5	8.2	3.3	
	1930–32	Lithuania	"	11.5	—	—	
	1935–41	Hungary	"	11.6	—	—	
	1931–32	Poland	"	11.7	—	—	
	1946–55	Sweden	"	11.7	8.6	3.2	
	1943–48	Switzerland	"	11.7	8.1	3.6	
	1946–55	Holland	"	11.9	8.1	3.7	
	1935–39	Bulgaria	"	11.9	—	—	
	1946–54	Norway	"	12.1	8.3	3.8	
	1949–55	Italy	"	12.3	8.6	3.7	
	1950–55	East Germany	"	12.4	9.1	3.3	
	1955	Yugoslavia	"	12.6	—	—	
	1931–33	Czechoslovakia	"	13.2	9.8	3.4	
	1931–38	Greece	"	13.8	10.9	2.9	
	1946–55	Denmark	"	14.2	—	—	
	1935–37	Finland	"	14.6	—	—	
	1935–37	Estonia	"	15.1	—	—	
	1936–38	Rumania	"	15.6	—	—	
	1935–38	Latvia	"	16.3	—	—	
Registrar-General (1958)	1938–56	England and Wales	"	12.3	8.8	3.5	
	1963–69	", ", "	"	11.4	—	—	At least one twin surviving
Statistical Bulletin of the Metropolitan Life	1950–57	USA	White population statistics	10.1	—	—	
			Negro	13.4	—	—	

Reference		Source				
	India and Pakistan					
Bulmer (1970)	Ahmedabad	Hospital statistics	12.9	7.6	5.3	225 twins
	Bangalore	"	10.2	7.3	2.9	493 twins
	Baroda	"	8.7	6.2	2.5	118 twins
	Bombay	"	11.1	6.8	4.3	1643 twins
Stevenson et al. (1966)	Bombay	"	12.2	7.2	5.0	490 twins
Bulmer (1970)	Calcutta	"	11.4	8.1	3.3	876 twins
Stevenson et al. (1966)	Calcutta	"	13.8	11.0	2.8	268 twins
Bulmer (1970)	Dibrugarh	"	10.5	7.0	3.5	105 twins
	Hyderabad	"	12.9	7.9	5.0	258 twins
	Lahore	"	23.3	15.5	7.8	108 twins
	Lucknow	"	13.2	8.0	5.2	109 twins
	Nagpur	"	17.5	11.1	6.4	164 twins
	Patna	"	17.4	11.2	6.2	115 twins
	Trivandrum	"	16.9	9.0	7.9	278 twins
	Visakhapatnam	"	13.2	8.5	4.7	361 twins
	Africa					
Bulmer (1960)	Ibadan (Nigeria)	Yoruba	45	42	4	603 twins
Knox and Morley (1960)	Ilesha (Nigeria)	Yoruba	54	49	5	158 twins
Nylander (1969)	Igbo-Ora (Nigeria)	Yoruba	46	42	4	177 twins
Cox (1963)	East (Nigeria)	Ibo	33	23	10	109 twins
Jeffreys (1953)	South (Nigeria)	Ibo	27	22	5	90 twins
	Natal	Zulu	28	21	7	116 twins
Ross (1952)	Bechuanaland	Tswana	18	10	8	87 twins
	Zimbabwe	Mashona	29	27	2	100 twins
	Asia					
Millis (1959)	Singapore	Chinese hospital	10.9	4.2	6.7	
Morton (1955)	Japan	Population statistics	4.3	1.3	3.0	
		Nagasaki & Hiroshima				

Table 2.2. The sex ratio in multiple births. From Bulmer (1970) by permission of the author and Oxford University Press

Country	Single	Twin	Triplet
England and Wales	0.515	0.508 ± 0.001	0.480 ± 0.009
France	0.514	0.506 ± 0.001	0.471 ± 0.009
Italy	0.515	0.508 ± 0.001	0.487 ± 0.008
U.S.A., white	0.514	0.507 ± 0.001	0.498 ± 0.006
U.S.A., negro	0.507	0.501 ± 0.001	0.502 ± 0.012
Japan	0.519	0.520 ± 0.004	0.515 ± 0.041

vulnerable male still further. Indeed in the most hazardous of all intrauterine environments for twins—the single amniotic sac—the sex ratio is very low (see p.66).

MZ and DZ Twins

The proportion of like- to unlike-sexed twins in a given population can be used to calculate the number of MZ and DZ twins. This is the basis for Weinberg's differential method. Weinberg (1902) reasoned that as the sex of each DZ twin is independently determined then there must be equal numbers of like- and unlike-sexed DZ twins. The number of MZ pairs must, therefore, be the excess of like-sexed over unlike-sexed pairs. Similarly the number of DZ pairs would be twice the number of unlike sex.

Thus the MZ and DZ twinning rates in a population may be calculated by the formulae

$$MZ = \frac{(L - U)}{N}$$

$$DZ = \frac{2U}{N}$$

where L and U are the number of like- and unlike-sexed twin maternities in a total sample of N maternities.

This does not allow for a sex ratio with the slightly higher incidence of males but apparently this minor discrepancy makes little difference to the overall figure (Bulmer 1970). Indeed, recent studies using elaborate methods of determining zygosity have reaped remarkably similar results.

MZ TWINS

MZ twins arise from the splitting of a zygote during the first 14 days after fertilization. At delivery correct identification of the placental membranes gives a good indication as to the stage of development at which this occurred (see p.72).

An MZ twinning rate of 3–4 per 1000 maternities appears to be constant worldwide and there are no factors which have yet been definitely associated with MZ twinning. Some workers have found a slight increase with maternal age (Bulmer 1970; Inouye and Imaizumi 1981) but this has not been confirmed by others (Nylander 1975c). In general all women appear to have the same chance of producing MZ twins and, unlike mothers of DZ twins, having had one set their risk of having another in a subsequent pregnancy is not increased. Having said that, there does now seem to be incontrovertible evidence of an occasional example of familial MZ twinning (Harvey et al. 1977; Segreti et al. 1978). Shapiro et al. (1978) describe a family with four sets of MZ twins in which the twinning gene appears to be carried by both males and females.

Nevertheless in epidemiological studies it has been shown repeatedly that families with MZ twins do not have larger numbers of twin relatives than expected and that the MZ twinning rate is independent of race (Morton 1962). Unless a mother of MZ twins has a strong history of MZ twins in the family she can be told that her chances of having twins again are not increased.

As implied, the causes of MZ twinning are unknown. Some believe it to be a form of congenital malformation caused by a developmental arrest early in embryonic life before tissue differentiation has begun (Stockard 1921). The global uniformity of the human MZ twinning rate may be due to the relative constancy of an intrauterine environment. In the less stable embryonic environment of an egg (a trout's in Stockard's case) it has been shown that twinning can be increased by depriving the egg of oxygen and warmth (Stockard 1921).

The increased incidence of congenital malformations in MZ twins may give support to this theory. On the other hand the malformations could be secondary to the MZ twinning process itself in that monochorionic placentation may well provide less favourable conditions for development. It remains to be shown whether congenital malformations are more common in monochorionic than dichorionic MZ twins (see p.48).

DZ TWINS

DZ twins result from the fertilization of two separately released ova. The number of DZ twin births can therefore be affected by the frequency of double ovulation, by sperm activity or by the rate of abortion (see p.32). The first is probably of the most import although the role of sperm activity may have been underestimated (James 1978).

Superfecundation and Superfetation

When two babies of apparently different ethnic origin were born in the same maternity, superfecundation (the conception of twins as a result of two coital acts in the same menstrual cycle) was suspected (Archer 1810). Different paternities have since been confirmed by blood grouping in several cases (Geyer 1940; Gedda 1961; Sorgo 1973) and more recently by HLA typing (Terasaki et al. 1978). Many others have been falsely suspected as Mauriceau (1721) indicates: '... another woman, who likewise had two children—the one like her husband, and the other like the gallant. But this does not prove superfoetation because sometimes different imaginations can cause the same effect'.

Further evidence of superfecundation is provided by the discordance for teratogenic malformations sometimes seen in DZ twins. If the twins are at different stages of development at the time of the teratogenic insult it follows that they were probably conceived at different times (see p.57).

Not surprisingly, in our monogamous society, the frequency of superfecundation is unknown.

It used to be thought, on the grounds of differences in birth weight, that twins were often conceived in separate menstrual cycles—superfetation. But weight is, of course, a poor indicator of gestational age. Even, indeed particularly, MZ twins may have large intrapair weight discrepancies. If superfetation occurs in man it is rare; Rhine and Nance (1976) however, describe an interesting family which, they suggest, has a dominant gene for superfetation. In four generations six pairs of twins (at least three of unlike sex) were born with marked weight discrepancies and in five pairs the smaller twin died in the perinatal period.

Causes of DZ Twinning

No single cause of DZ twinning is known but, unlike MZ twinning, at least some of the associated factors have been recognized. It has been estimated that between 11 and 27% of Caucasian women are twin-prone (Wyshak and White 1965*b*), a far greater number than those who actually produce twins. Lazar et al. (1981) have devised a scoring system by which they can predict the probability of a twin pregnancy for a particular woman. For their calculation they use seven maternal characteristics which they found to be associated with twinning (see p.27). We are still, however, far from being able to predict accurately which women will have twins and research on this subject is much needed.

Genetic and Racial

It is well known that twins 'run in families' but there are still many falsely held beliefs, such as that twins usually occur in alternate generations.

Family studies have now shown that the genetic determinant for twinning comes directly through the female line (Weinberg 1902; Bulmer 1960; White and Wyshak 1964; Nylander 1975*a*) but may well not be expressed in each generation. Early reports of an increased incidence of twins on the paternal side of the family (Davenport 1927; Curtius 1928; Greulich 1934) are now thought to have been due to under-reporting of singletons (Nylander 1975*a*). Restriction of the carrier gene to females was also suggested by Morton's (1962) study of nearly 180 000 children in Hawaii which showed that in inter-racial marriages DZ twinning rates depend on the mother's race.

It appears that the gene concerned influences gonadotrophin production. Nylander (1973) found that in three groups of Nigerian (Yoruba) mothers, one with singletons, another with one set of twins each and a third with two sets each, there was a positive correlation between serum FSH (follicle stimulating hormone) levels and twinning, with a difference between each of the three groups. Similarly Nigerian mothers of singletons had higher levels of FSH (Nylander 1978) than mothers of singletons in Japan, where it is well established that there are particularly low rates of twinning (Soma et al. 1975).

No amount of bias in reporting could account for the vastly disparate twinning rates found in different ethnic groups throughout the world. The chance of a woman from the Yoruba tribe in Nigeria having twins is about eight times that of one from Taiwan (Ping and Chin 1967) and five times that of most Caucasians. Indeed, similar disparities are found in inter-racial populations where the accuracy of twin statistics in all groups is probably similar (Morton 1962). In the United States the non-white population has a consistently higher twinning rate than the whites (Bulmer 1958*b*) although not as high as most African groups. This may be due to the introduction of some Caucasian genes by inter-racial marriages or to environmental differences.

All negro races have a relatively high twinning rate but there is still considerable variation between ethnic groups, as Nylander found in his study of the various tribes in Nigeria (Nylander 1971*a*; Nylander and Corney 1977). Unusually high rates have also been found in some isolated Caucasian groups such as those in the remote Finnish islands of Åland (Eriksson and Fellman 1973). The high incidence amongst isolated groups is likely to be the result of endogamy. The increasing number of immigrant marriage partners in Åland has been reflected in a falling twinning rate since the beginning of this century (Eriksson and Fellman 1973).

Theoretically both the familial and the racial determinants of DZ twinning could be essentially environmental. In support of this idea is Nylander's finding of a much lower incidence of twins in Yoruba women living in towns than in rural villages. This could not be accounted for by the age or parity differences alone. Nylander suggests that the traditional diet of this tribe may contain some hormone stimulating substance, possibly in the yam, which is eaten less by those living an urban and therefore more Westernized life (Nylander 1978, 1979). However, Morton's (1962) findings in Hawaii contradict a purely environmental determinant as in inter-racial marriages both parents (presumably) share the same environment, including diet. It is likely that both genetics and environment play a part in DZ twinning.

Maternal Age and Parity
The elderly mother with an already large family is the one most likely (and often least eager) to have twins. Many authors (Anderson 1956; Bulmer 1959*a*; Millis 1959; Eriksson and Fellman 1967; Nylander 1975*c*; Elwood 1978) have reported that the incidence of twins increases with age, reaching a peak at 35–39 years (Fig. 2.1). Nylander (1975*c*) suggests that this is due to increasing ovarian activity until the late thirties. Thereafter the graafian follicles become exhausted as the menopause approaches.

Earlier studies related to Caucasian populations but Nylander (1971*b*, 1975*c*) has found the same pattern in Nigeria except that here the peak is reached earlier, at 30–34 years. Women start childbearing earlier in West Africa and it may be that the ovaries

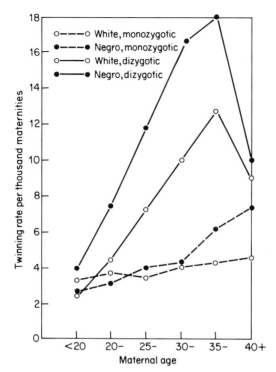

Fig. 2.1. The twinning rate among American whites and negroes, by maternal age. From Bulmer (1958*b*) by permission of the author and editors of *Annals of Human Genetics* and Cambridge University Press.

then reach maximal activity earlier than Caucasians. DZ twinning rates increase with parity independent of maternal age (Bulmer 1970; Nylander 1975*c*; Fig. 2.2). This is scarcely surprising as both DZ twins and a large family are signs of high fertility. Other indications that mothers of twins conceive easily is the high twinning rate amongst illegitimate births (particularly in women over 25 years) (Eriksson and Fellman 1967; Campbell et al. 1974), as well as those conceived in the first 3 months of marriage (Bulmer 1959*a*; Allen 1981). There was a rush of twin births in the United States in 1946 and this was probably due to a twinning tendency in those women who conceived most quickly following the return of the fathers at the end of World War II (Allen and Schachter 1970). However, in the last three instances coital rates are likely to be high and it could be that more frequent sexual intercourse could account for the high twinning rate by increasing the chances of super-fecundation (James 1972*a*).

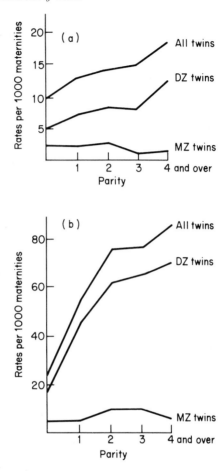

Fig. 2.2. Influence of parity on the incidence of twinning in (a) Aberdeen, and (b) Nigeria. From Nylander (1975*c*) by permission of the author and W.B. Saunders Co. Ltd.

Maternal Height and Weight

More tall women than small have twins (Anderson 1956; Campbell et al. 1974; Corney et al. 1979). Similarly weight appears to have a positive correlation with DZ twinning (Campbell et al. 1974). Both height and weight are indices of nutrition; Bulmer (1959*b*) found that in countries where there was severe shortage of food in World War II such as France, the Netherlands and Norway, twinning rates fell whereas in countries in which there was no undernourishment such as Sweden and Denmark they were unchanged during the war.

Other Maternal Factors

Women who have borne twins tend to differ from mothers of singletons in their menstrual and reproductive histories. It has been found that women with irregular menstrual cycles are less likely to have twins (Hemon et al. 1979) and that there is a positive correlation between twinning and both early menarche (Skerlj 1939; Wyshak 1981) and short menstrual cycles (Wyshak 1981). Likewise Wyshak (1978) found that mothers of twins have an earlier natural menopause than mothers of singletons.

It appears that the introduction of hormone-suppressing agents for contraception may well have affected the pattern of DZ twinning. Whereas there appears to be an increased chance of a multiple pregnancy immediately after stopping oral contraception, probably due to a rebound effect on the previously suppressed pituitary hormones (Rothman 1977; Bracken 1979), the overall chances of a multiple pregnancy in women who have previously used oral contraception are less than in those who have never taken hormone suppressing drugs (Rothman 1977; Hemon et al. 1979).

Social Class

Studies of both Caucasians and Africans have shown that twins are more common in lower social classes (Smith 1966; Nylander 1971*b*). This is probably due to their propensity for having large families.

Seasonal Variation

Timonen and Carpen (1968) reported a marked seasonal variation in twinning rates and suggested that the higher rate of twin conceptions in the summer months in Finland might be due to the increased hours of daylight. Several other authors (Edwards 1938; Knox and Morley 1960; Kamimura 1976; Elwood 1978) have reported seasonal variations in twinning. Some have related these to climatic conditions in their countries but no regular pattern emerges.

Secular Trends in Twinning Rates

In recent years many developed countries including the USA, many parts of Western Europe, Australia, New Zealand, Japan (James 1972*b*), Hungary (Czeizel and Acsárdi, 1971), Poland (Rola-Janicki 1974) and Canada (Elwood 1973), have reported a fall in their twinning rates—the oft quoted figure of 1 in 80 deliveries in the UK is now outdated and this should be revised to 1 in 100. Where this decline has been analysed it appears to be confined to DZ twins. In most countries it started in the 1950s and is continuing. In the USA, however, it occurred earlier and the rate is now steady (Jeanneret and Macmahon 1962), possibly because the trend has been counteracted by ovulation-stimulating drugs (James 1978).

The cause of the fall in twinning rates is unknown. Earlier age of childbearing and smaller families are not the full explanation (James 1975); use of oral contraceptives and pesticides has been suggested, so has the rise in levels of air, water and soil pollution (Eriksson et al. 1976). Recently James (1978) offered a theory that reduced sperm activity may be responsible as there is evidence, at least in the USA, that sperm counts have fallen in recent years (Nelson and Bunge 1974; Rehan et al. 1975).

From developing countries we have only the reports from parts of Nigeria (Nylander 1975c). Here the rates are still increasing, possibly due to improved nutrition.

DETERMINATION OF ZYGOSITY

Whatever the reason, most parents of twins are anxious to learn the zygosity of their twins as soon as possible. Few are satisfied by the assurance that this is likely to become apparent by the children's second birthday. Quite apart from the advantages to medical and scientific research this is ample reason for determining as accurately as practicable the zygosity of all newborn twins.

Where their sex differs there is of course no problem. Taking placentation also into account the zygosity of over half of Caucasian twins can be determined in the delivery room.

Sex

One-third of all twins are of unlike sex and all these must be DZ, with the exception of an extremely rare case of heterokaryotypic chromosomal anomaly (see p.50).

Placentation

For many years it was believed that all MZ twins had a single chorion. Indeed some medical textbooks still categorically state this and some paediatricians still appear to believe them. Parents may still present their indistinguishable 4- or 5-year-old twins and declare that they are fraternal because they had two placentae.

It is now known that those MZ twins whose zygote has divided before the sixth day after fertilization, have separate chorions. This, as well as the method of examination of placental membranes, will be discussed more fully in Chapter 4. Suffice is to say here that only two-thirds of MZ twins will have monochorionic placentae. In these a definite diagnosis of monozygosity can be made as no convincing report of a monochorionic placenta in a DZ pregnancy has been offered.

Nearly half of Caucasian twins have dichorionic placentae and are of like sex. For these, other lines of zygosity determination are necessary.

Physical Features

In older children and adults physical features are a relatively good means of establishing zygosity (Cohen et al. 1975; Kasriel and Eaves 1976). In a study of 200 pairs of Swedish twins Cederlof et al. (1961) found that out of 72 who affirmed in a reply to a mailed questionnaire that they had grown up 'as alike as two peas', 71 were subsequently found to be alike for the five blood groups tested. But appearances are of little help in newborn twins. Intrauterine influences may well be stronger than genetic ones particularly in cases of the fetofetal transfusion syndrome (see p.46), when MZ twins may have large intrapair weight discrepancies.

Ear form has been suggested as a useful guide (Dahlberg 1926) but comparing two tiny ears is not easy. Nor is the comparison of finger and palm prints. The ridge count on fingers is thought to be genetically determined and thus the counts can give some indication of zygosity (Smith and Penrose 1955; Holt 1968). So can the sum of the left and right maximal ATD palmar angles (Holt 1968). As the overlap between MZ and DZ is considerable these methods are only useful as adjuncts to others.

Blood Grouping

As MZ twins are derived from one zygote they must be alike for all genetically determined characters whereas DZ twins originating from two zygotes are no more alike than siblings. The most useful genetically determined characteristics to study are those with a

Table 2.3. Biochemical genetic markers used at the MRC Human Genetics Unit, University College, London, in the determination of zygosity in newborn twins. Relative chances in favour of dizygosity are given for each genetically determined character. From Corney and Robson (1975) by permission of the authors and W.B. Saunders Co. Ltd.

Enzyme or serum protein system		Twin pair of like phenotype	Relative chance in favour of dizygosity
Tissue enzymes typed on placenta			
Placental alkaline phosphatase		1	0.7006
Pl		2-1	0.5606
		2	0.3856
		3-1	0.4678
		3	0.2938
		3-2	0.3417
Phosphoglucomutase, locus 3		1	0.7569
PGM_3		2-1	0.5962
		2	0.3969
Red cell enzymes			
Acid phosphatase, locus 1		A	0.4624
ACP_1		BA	0.5937
		B	0.6320
		CA	0.3615
		CB	0.4248
		C	0.2756
Phosphoglucomutase, locus 1		1	0.7788
PGM_1		2-1	0.5899
		2	0.3813
Adenylate kinase		1	0.9555
AK		2-1	0.5215
		2	0.2730
Adenosine deaminase		1	0.9409
ADA		2-1	0.5282
		2	0.2809
Esterase-D		1	0.9054
$ES-D$		2-1	0.5438
		2	0.3008
Glutamic-pyruvic transaminase		1	0.5646
GPT		2-1	0.6250
		2	0.5588
Serum proteins			
Group-specific component		1	0.7569
Gc		2-1	0.5962
		2	0.3969
α_1-antitrypsin		M	0.9555
Pi	*S or other non-M types	MS*	0.5215
		S*	0.2730
Haptoglobin (sometimes developed		1-1	0.4761
Hp	in the newborn)	2-1	0.6178
		2-2	0.6561

simple mode of inheritance and commonly occurring variation such as blood groups.

Typing of blood groups—or, more accurately, red cell antigens—is the most commonly used and practical means of determining zygosity. ABO, rhesus and MNSs can be measured in any blood transfusion unit and all can be obtained from cord blood. More recently other such genetic markers, namely red cell enzymes, serum proteins and tissue enzymes (in particular placental alkaline phosphatase) as well as those demonstrated by histocompatibility testing have been added to the repertoire. But the typing of these is available in fewer units—usually those specializing in biochemical genetics.

Table 2.3 shows the biochemical genetic markers used in determining zygosity at the MRC Human Biochemical Genetics Unit, Galton Laboratory, University College, London.

Clearly if any marker differs the twins must be DZ. In practice if only one is different out of a large number examined a repeat

Table 2.4. An example of the determination of the chances of dizygosity in a pair of twins alike for all blood group and biochemical markers and of the most common phenotype at all loci, using the tables of Smith and Penrose (1955) and Race and Sanger (1975). From Corney and Robson (1975) by permission of the authors and W.B. Saunders Co. Ltd.

Marker system		Phenotype	Relative chance of dizygosity for a particular system	Relative chance of monozygosity for a particular system
	Initial odds		0.7000	0.3
Sex		Female	0.5000	1.0
ABO		A	0.6945	1.0
MNSs		MS	0.5161	1.0
Rh		R_1r	0.5400	1.0
Kell		K–	0.9548	1.0
Secretor		Sec	0.8681	1.0
Duffy		Fy(a+)	0.8099	1.0
Kidd		Jk(a+)	0.8616	1.0
Dombrock		Do(a+)	0.8094	1.0
Xg		Xg(a+)	0.9573	1.0
Pl		1	0.7006	1.0
PGM_3		1	0.7569	1.0
ACP_1		B	0.6320	1.0
ADA		1	0.9409	1.0
ES-D		1	0.9054	1.0
GPT		2-1	0.6250	1.0
Gc		1	0.7569	1.0
Pi		M	0.9555	1.0
Combined chance after testing			0.0056	0.3
Chance of dizygosity = 0.0056/0.3056 = 0.0183				

P, Yt and *Hp* have not been used as they are not fully developed in the newborn, and *Lu, PGM₁* and *AK* because they are linked to *Sec, Rh* and *ABO* respectively.

examination on a fresh blood sample is advisable to exclude a technical error. Monozygosity can never be proven by marker testing but the probability increases with the number tested and an exact probability can be calculated (Table 2.4). This is more precise if the parent's blood types and race are known. Values in favour of monozygosity of over 99.5% may be reached. Without such information on the parents estimations are made according to the gene frequency in the particular ethnic group and tables of the relevant data are available (Race and Sanger 1975).

Intertwin acceptance of skin grafts is often stated to be the ultimate confirmation of monozygosity. The situation is however complex, incompletely understood and therefore difficult to quantify (Corney and Robson 1975). Skin grafting in twins as a means of determining zygosity is in any case both unjustified and unethical, particularly in the newborn.

Methods of zygosity determination are comprehensively reviewed by Corney and Robson (1975).

3. Multiple Pregnancy

A mother may learn that she is expecting two babies as early as the 6th week of her pregnancy. On the other hand she may have no suspicion until after the birth of the first baby. At whatever stage the twin is discovered most parents have a time of shock followed by readjustment; it is clearly better that this process be completed before the mother has to look after the two babies. Several mothers have described their difficulties in bonding to two fetuses when they had already developed a deeply felt relationship with what they thought was one baby. This is particularly true when twins are discovered only in the third trimester.

The medical hazards, as well as the practical and psychological problems, which may confront a mother of undiagnosed twins, are now well known. In centres where ultrasound scanning is not routinely practised there may be a place for selective screening of predictably high-risk cases such as a mother with a family history of twins (Michels and Riccardi 1978). Other criteria for screening can be deduced from Chapter 2.

As a result of their study of a large number of French mothers of twins Lazar et al. (1981) suggested a scale for preconceptional prediction of twins using six maternal features—age, parity, twins in her family, regularity of menses and blood groups O or A.

DIAGNOSIS

Before the advent of screening with ultrasound scanners an unexpected second baby was not uncommon and in some centres 50%

of mothers went into labour before twins had been diagnosed (Farooqui et al. 1973; MacGillivray 1975*a*; Grennert et al. 1976). In those pregnancies where twins were detected diagnosis rested on clinical suspicion followed by radiological confirmation. An inappropriately large uterus, an unusually rapid weight gain or the palpation of multiple fetal parts are all possible indications for an abdominal x-ray. In obstetric units with no routine screening procedures most multiple pregnancies are not diagnosed until after the 30th week—long after the time at which a mother should be having special care, supervision and extra rest.

There is a range of cheaper and more readily available methods of screening for multiple pregnancy than ultrasound which may be more appropriate first lines of investigation in some centres. These include measurements of maternal serum alphafetoprotein (AFP),

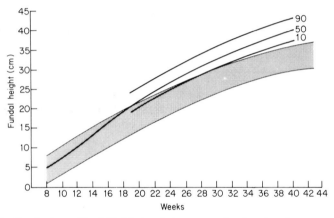

Fig. 3.1. Centile chart of fundal height in relation to gestational age in twin pregnancy. The shaded area shows the normal range for singleton pregnancy. From Leroy et al. (1982) by permission of the authors.

human choriogonadotrophin, and human placental lactogen (HPL). In developing countries the most efficient method of detecting a multiple pregnancy is likely to be an accurate clinical measurement, such as the fundal height. Leroy et al. (1982) found that 90% of multiple pregnancies had a fundal height above the 90th centile for a single pregnancy by the 20th week and 98% by the 28th week (Fig. 3.1).

Alphafetoprotein

Maternal serum AFP is routinely measured in many antenatal clinics as a screening test for fetal neural tube defects. Two fetuses increase the total AFP production and this is reflected in the maternal serum. One study showed that nearly 80% of maternal AFP levels in multiple pregnancies were above the 90th centile for a single pregnancy (Knight et al. 1981). Thus a mother with a raised serum AFP may have a period of intense anxiety only relieved by the discovery that her raised AFP is due to nothing worse than twins. AFP values in twin pregnancies, however, vary over a wide range so that some cases will still fall well within the normal limits for a single pregnancy.

Human Placental Lactogen and Human Choriogonadotrophin

Maternal serum HPL estimations between the 29th and 30th weeks of gestation may indicate a multiple pregnancy. Mägiste et al. (1976) found that all of 32 mothers of twins had serum levels of more than 5.0 μg/ml in contrast to only 10% of single pregnancies.

Similar trends have been observed by other workers (Grennert et al. 1976; Merkatz 1979) but it is yet to be shown whether this test can be reliably applied earlier in pregnancy.

Jovanovic et al. (1977) give an encouraging preliminary report on the value of serum human gonadotrophin levels in detecting twins early in pregnancy. They found that the levels were already higher in multiple than single pregnancies at the time of the pregnancy confirmation test only 4 or 5 weeks after the last menstrual period.

Ultrasound

With routine screening of all pregnancies for twins some centres now approach 100% detection rate (Morrison et al. 1970; Grennert et al. 1976) and the average stage of pregnancy at which the diagnosis is made is substantially earlier. In one unit the average time of diagnosis fell from 33 weeks to 19 weeks over a 6-year period following the introduction of ultrasound screening (Grennert et al. 1976; Figs 3.2 and 3.3). However 12–16 weeks—the stage of pregnancy at which most routine scanning is carried out—is not the easiest time to detect twins and in less experienced hands the second fetus may quite often be missed. In one study one-fifth of all multiple pregnancies in which an ultrasound scan was carried out had at least one false negative report (Jarvis 1979). Some patients

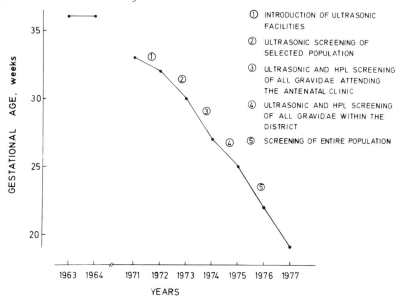

Fig. 3.2. Average gestational age at diagnosis of twin pregnancy in relation to introduction of diagnostic facilities. By permission of L. Grennert (1982, personal communication).

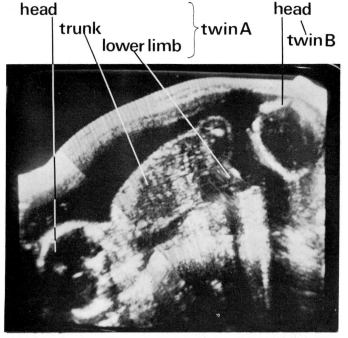

Fig. 3.3. Ultrasonic scan at 24 weeks' gestation showing two fetuses. By permission of Dr Valerie Farr.

have had three scans and still been surprised by a second baby at delivery.

A multiple pregnancy can be diagnosed as early as 5 weeks; a quintuplet pregnancy was detected at 9 weeks (Campbell and Dewhurst 1970). With these very early diagnoses the question is whether to tell the parents immediately and risk a later disappointment (see p.157). This risk is much higher than generally recognized. There is evidence that in 50% or more of twin pregnancies one fetus is lost (Robinson and Caines 1977)—the 'vanishing twin syndrome' (Fig. 3.4). Indeed Levi (1976) found that only 29% of

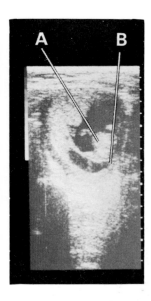

Fig. 3.4. Ultrasonic scan of twin pregnancy at 13 weeks' gestation showing one normal fetus (A) and one empty sac (B). Vaginal blood loss occurred at 12 weeks. By permission of Dr Valerie Farr.

twin pregnancies diagnosed before the 10th week ended up with two live babies. The majority of mothers had one full-term baby. Schneider et al. (1978) confirmed these findings and made an interesting observation in relation to ovulation-induced twin pregnancies. In the 11 cases in which clomiphene had been taken ovular resorption occurred in seven whereas in the 12 pregnancies induced by gonadotropins all resulted in the delivery of two babies.

X-rays

X-rays, the mainstay of diagnosis of multiple pregnancy in the past, are much less often used now, as they are being superseded by

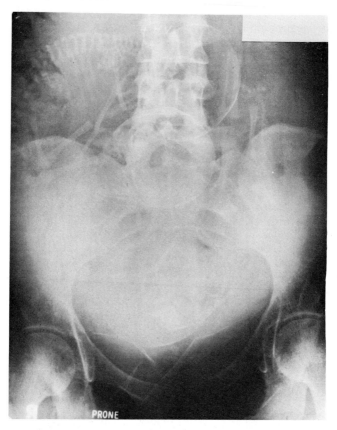

Fig. 3.5. X-ray showing triplets. By permission of J. Malvern.

ultrasound scans. There are, however, still times when x-rays are needed, for example when ultrasound scanning gives an equivocal result or if more than two fetuses are suspected (Fig. 3.5). An x-ray is also indicated in the case of fetal malposition or suspected fetal bony abnormalities (Fig. 3.6). Radiography for assessing the position of the fetuses has now been largely superseded by ultrasound.

ABORTION

Spontaneous abortions of twins are often missed as, in many of the earlier cases, the fetuses are not distinguished. It follows that figures on the incidence of twin abortions should be interpreted with caution. Incidence of up to 20% have been recorded but in two large studies of approximately 2000 abortions each the incidence of twins was only 1.2% (Javert 1957) and 0.3% (Benirschke and Driscoll 1967). However, in a more recent study in which 1939 spontaneously aborted embryos and fetuses were examined in

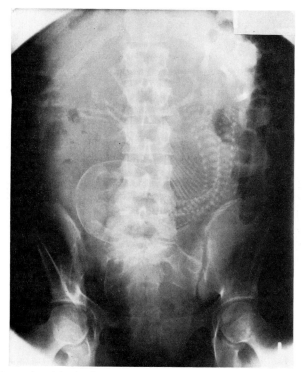

Fig. 3.6. X-ray of conjoined twins.

detail the incidence of twin abortions was 3%—approximately three times greater than would be expected (Livingston and Poland 1980). The authors distinguished between embryos (less than 30 mm crown–rump length) and fetuses and found the same increase in both groups when compared with singletons.

Amongst aborted twins there is a striking preponderance of monochorionic twins (Livingston and Poland 1980). Disturbances of the fetofetoplacental circulation are probably responsible for many abortions in this group. Out of the 26 fetuses examined

Livingston and Poland found definite evidence of the fetofetal transfusion syndrome in eight. Javert (1957) found that there were relatively fewer malformed fetuses amongst twins and attributed this to the disproportionately high incidence of circulatory disturbances. Perhaps surprisingly Livingston and Poland did not confirm this finding. They found a similar proportion of malformations amongst both twin embryos and fetuses as singletons.

The death of just one fetus, which may or may not be aborted, is quite common. This is shown by the relatively high incidence of twins found in first-trimester ultrasound scans (see p.31) compared with the number of twins actually delivered. Similarly, on routine ultrasound screening, it is not unusual to find an empty second gestational sac. In one large study this occurred in 0.8% of all pregnancies (Ramzin et al. 1982). Evidence of a blighted twin may also be seen in some cases of first-trimester bleeding with continuation of a normal single pregnancy (Finberg and Birnholz 1979).

COMPLICATIONS AND MANAGEMENT OF MULTIPLE PREGNANCY

The high perinatal mortality associated with twinning is largely due to complications of pregnancy such as premature onset of labour, fetal intrauterine growth retardation and difficulties of delivery. The management of multiple pregnancy is thus concerned with the prevention, early detection, and treatment of these complications.

The role of some measures (to promote fetal growth and prevent premature onset of labour) such as bedrest, cervical cerclage and β-sympathomimetic drugs remains controversial (Weekes et al. 1977*b*). Discussions on these and other aspects of management are beyond the scope of this book and the reader is referred to *Human Multiple Reproduction* (MacGillivray et al. 1975) and to textbooks on obstetrics.

Pre-eclamptic Toxaemia

Pre-eclampsia, an important complication of pregnancy, is generally recognized to occur more often in multiple pregnancy. The actual incidences reported inevitably vary according to diagnostic criteria. Several authors have found at least a threefold increase compared with singletons (Guttmacher 1939; Bender 1952) but the increase in incidence of the severe form may be higher still (MacGillivray 1958). Pre-eclampsia is characteristically a disorder of primagravidae but MacGillivray (1958) found that the chances of the severe form developing in a second (twin) pregnancy if the first (single) had been normal were 130 times that in a second single pregnancy.

Studies of multiple pregnancies give no convincing support to the theory of an immunological basis for pre-eclamptic toxaemia. Were it so, the disease should be more common in DZ pregnancies than in MZ. However, Campbell et al. (1977), in their study of over 300 multiple pregnancies, found no higher incidence of either the mild or the severe form of pre-eclampsia in mothers of DZ twins.

Polyhydramnios

The volume of amniotic fluid present in multiple pregnancy is particularly difficult to assess as the bulk of two fetuses can give the false impression of an increased amount of fluid. As with pre-eclampsia differences in criteria largely account for the varying incidences reported and as amniotic fluid is rarely accurately measured it is usually a subjective diagnosis. With these reservations, however, comparisons within a single centre are probably valid and most authors agree that polyhydramnios is more common in multiple pregnancy and that there is a high perinatal mortality associated with it. Law (1967) found that twins from a multiple pregnancy complicated by polyhydramnios had almost three times the risk of a perinatal death as those from pregnancies without increased volumes of amniotic fluid. Perhaps surprisingly this increase in the occurrence of polyhydramnios affects DZ as much as MZ pregnancies (Nylander and MacGillivray 1975*b*).

At least some of the MZ cases of polyhydramnios are the results of the fetofetal transfusion syndrome (see p.46) where the recipient twin's hypervolaemia results in polyuria and a consequent increase in amniotic fluid. Kloosterman (1963) suggested that the hypervolaemia, in turn, is due to an increase in maternofetal transfer of fluid in response to high fetal plasma proteins. The fetofetal transfusion syndrome, together with cases secondary to congenital malformations, at least partially explain the increased perinatal mortality associated with polyhydramnios (Tow 1959; Farooqui et al. 1973).

The high incidence of polyhydramnios in DZ pregnancies is harder to explain unless the increased intrauterine load somehow impedes the circulation and reabsorption of amniotic fluid.

The rare condition of acute polyhydramnios with its high fetal wastage appears to be confined to MZ twin pregnancies. Weir et al. (1979) found eight cases in over 30 000 deliveries. Two of these were in monoamniotic pregnancies and the remaining six were monochorionic diamniotic. All occurred in the second trimester between the 21st and 28th weeks and ended in a premature delivery within a few days. Apart from a pair of campomelic dwarfs the fetuses were normal, which suggests that a disturbance in the fetoplacental circulation is the most likely cause.

Acute polyhydramnios is a rapidly progressive disorder precipitating a premature delivery within a few days of onset. Spontaneous abatement seems to occur only if one fetus dies (Bender 1952). Repeated amniocentesis to remove the fluid may prevent the onset of labour long enough to produce a viable baby. Bender's (1952) patient had eight taps over 7 weeks.

Other less serious complications occur in multiple as in single pregnancies but the symptoms are often more severe. Such a large uterine load may cause many symptoms including breathlessness, indigestion and backache. These can be distressing and worrying to a mother. Even if the discomfort cannot be alleviated she will feel much better if reassured that these symptoms are a normal, if unfortunate, part of a twin pregnancy.

Although the general management of a multiple pregnancy is rarely the concern of the paediatrician until the time for delivery is approaching, there are some aspects about which both obstetrician and patient may value his advice. Amniocentesis is one of these.

Amniocentesis

Amniocentesis presents a particular problem in multiple pregnancy (Hunter and Cox 1979). It is technically more difficult and dangerous. The risks of inducing an abortion are greater. In addition, the results may pose a far greater dilemma for parents of twins than singletons as the chances of both twins being abnormal are small. For these reasons some centres, such as Aberdeen, feel that amniocentesis in a twin pregnancy is contraindicated (D.M. Campbell 1982, personal communication).

Amniocentesis is now offered to many elderly mothers for the detection of chromosomal abnormalities and to others with a personal or family history of neural tube defects or some genetically determined disorder. A multiple pregnancy, however, alters the risks of some abnormalities. For instance, trisomy 21 is less common in twins whereas neural tube defects are more so. On the other hand concordance for neural tube defects, even in MZ twins, is unusual and Down's syndrome, although usually concordant in MZ twins, rarely affects both of a DZ pair (see p.50).

Although some centres report excellent results (Elias et al. 1980) others find it technically difficult to aspirate fluid from both amniotic sacs. Some parents are thus faced with making a decision on the findings from only one specimen.

Many mothers who would not hesitate to have a pregnancy terminated for a single abnormal fetus could not agree if it meant the sacrifice of a normal baby at the same time. Yet the stress of knowingly carrying an abnormal fetus for the remainder of the pregnancy may have a terrible effect on the mother. For others their decision may depend on whether the affected child is likely to die at or soon after birth or survive as a burden to himself, his twin and his family for many years.

As children with anencephaly and the more severe forms of spina bifida die early in life many parents who would otherwise have accepted an amniocentesis to exclude these malformations may choose not to have the investigation in the presence of twins. Careful counselling to both parents on all these aspects is vital before proceeding to a diagnostic amniocentesis.

Selective intrauterine death of the abnormal fetus, either by cardiac puncture, or by injection of an air embolus into the umbilical vein has now been effected on several occasions (Aberg et al. 1978; Kerenyi and Chitkara 1981). If this becomes more general practice the horror of aborting a normal fetus will be removed. The parents, however, will need a great deal of support and counselling throughout the pregnancy and, sometimes, for many years after (see Chapter 13).

PREPARATION FOR TWINS

For a mother expecting her first baby there are endless sources of advice and information. In addition, whether she likes it or not, she will be deluged with stories of experiences that others have been through before her. In contrast a mother who is told that she is having twins often knows no other mother of twins to whom she can turn with all the questions and worries that spring up. In one study only one of 23 mothers who heard that they were expecting twins, knew another mother of twins well enough to contact her (Bryan 1977*b*). At best these mothers are short of information; there is little literature readily available. At worst they are upset by misleading old wives' tales about the difficulties of twin labours and the frailty of twin children. All will have questions and fears; all too often these are not voiced, partly because of the discouraging bustle of the antenatal clinic. Both parents are in urgent need of support and information to cope with the prospect of an unplanned and, for some, unwelcome extra baby.

Emotional and practical support can best be provided by other mothers of twins. Few medical staff have the appropriate practical knowledge. Most areas in the UK now have a local parents of twins club, members of which are happy to make immediate contact with an expectant mother. Failing this the national Twins Clubs Association gives contact addresses in the area as well as providing literature on practical aspects of multiple pregnancy and the care of twin children. Similar organizations have been started in other countries (see Chapter 15).

Many mothers find that some equipment useful for one baby is inappropriate in duplicate. Much money can be saved by prior discussion with other mothers of twins. It is wise to discourage mothers from actually buying a twin pram before the babies are born and seen to be well. It is often possible to reserve a pram through shops or a second-hand one through the twins club. Should one or both babies die this expensive and painful reminder of the lost twin(s) is then avoided.

For the unexpected second baby the twins club can often provide all necessary equipment.

4. The Twin Fetus

From the moment of fertilization the development of the human fetus depends on the intrauterine environment. The twin fetus, however, is affected not only by these innumerable environmental factors but must also interact with a second fetus. At best it must compete for nutrition. At worst it may be severely, even lethally, damaged by the co-twin.

INTRAUTERINE GROWTH

It is no wonder that newborn twins tend to be smaller than singletons. The twin fetus has to share—often unequally—the maternal supply of nourishment and, in monochorionic twins, there is the additional handicap of an energy wasting 'third circulation' (see p.77).

Surprisingly, a fetus of a twin pregnancy does usually manage to grow at the same rate as a singleton for the first two trimesters (McKeown and Record 1952; Naeye et al. 1966, Fig. 4.1). The few that do not are likely to be the much lighter twins in grossly weight-discordant pairs (Crane et al. 1980).

From the 26–28th week onwards the rate of growth decreases in comparison to that of a singleton. The average weight of a newborn twin is about 800 g less than a singleton but if allowance is made for differences in gestational age the discrepancy is reduced to 500 g (Hemon et al. 1982). As a result of their study on over 2000 liveborn twins between 24 and 42 weeks gestation Naeye et al. (1966) produced the centile charts shown in Fig. 4.2. They found that monochorionic twins were, in general, lighter than dichorionic for the period of gestation and that their intrapair variation in weight was greater.

As in many animal species the growth of the human fetus is influenced by litter size and the deceleration in growth rate which occurs at about 36 weeks in singletons takes place correspondingly earlier in twins and higher multiple births. McKeown and Record (1952) suggest that this deceleration occurs when the total litter weight reaches a critical level—about 3 kg in man.

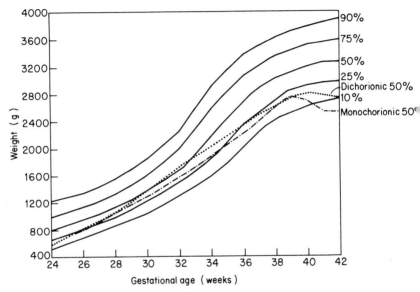

Fig. 4.1. Birth weights of live monochorionic and dichorionic twins compared with singletons. From Naeye et al. (1966) by permission of the authors and the editors of *Pediatrics*. Copyright American Academy of Pediatrics 1966.

The typical pattern of intrauterine growth of twins is similar to that of growth-retarded singletons in that the weight falls away disproportionately more than the occipitofrontal circumference or the length (Fenner et al. 1980). Factors associated with intrauterine growth retardation in singletons, such as maternal size and smoking, apply equally to twins (Hemon et al. 1982). There are of course additional, and partly unexplained, factors operating in a multiple pregnancy.

The mechanical restraint of uterine overcrowding seems unlikely to be a significant factor. The work of Morris et al. (1955) suggests that uteroplacental perfusion is reduced in multiple pregnancy.

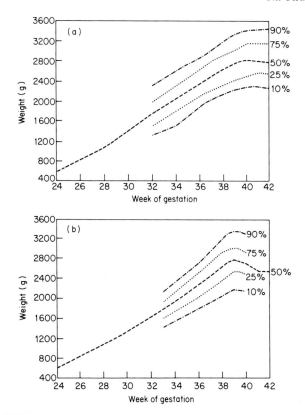

Fig. 4.2. Birth weights of live (a) dichorionic, and (b) monochorionic twins. From Naeye et al. (1966) by permission of the authors and the editors of *Pediatrics*. Copyright American Academy of Pediatrics 1966.

Indirect evidence of a reduced oxygen supply to the twin fetus is provided by the higher cord blood haemoglobin levels found in twins and also the fact that in twin pairs of discordant weight the smaller tends to have the higher haemoglobin level (Walker and Turnbull 1955; Clemetson 1956).

Zygosity

Even when allowance is made for length of gestation MZ twins are lighter than DZ. This difference in weight was originally attributed to the reduced efficiency of a monochorionic placenta. However, Corney et al. (1972), whilst confirming the findings of others of a weight discordance between the two types of twins, showed that this could not be explained by the effects of placentation (nor indeed by a number of other variables). That is to say that even MZ twins with two chorions and, therefore, separate circulations, were lighter than DZ. There was no obvious reason for this weight difference but the authors offered three possible explanations. The first was that the low weight could be related to events in early embryonic development when the cell mass is reduced by its division into two embryos. Secondly, the explanation may be immunological. The antigenic differences between DZ twins could beneficially affect intrauterine growth. Thirdly, maternal factors may play a part. The mothers of DZ twins are, on average, taller and their levels of hormones higher than mothers of MZ.

Placenta

The growth of the twin fetus is affected by the site of implantation of the placenta in the uterus (see p.73); the site of umbilical cord insertion into the placenta (see p.74); the absence of an umbilical artery (see p.75); and, in monochorionic twins, by the haemodynamic effects of the 'third circulation' (see p.76).

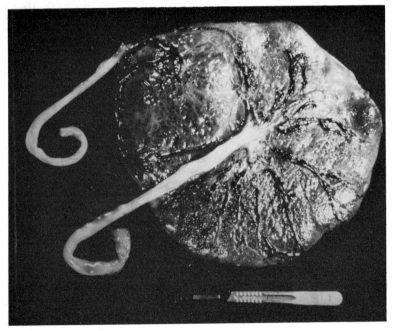

Fig. 4.3. Monochorionic placenta of infants shown in Fig. 4.4. with eccentric insertion of one umbilical cord.

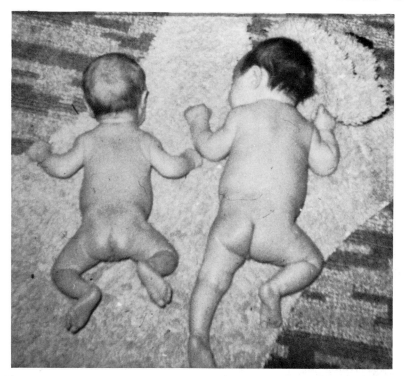

Fig. 4.4. MZ twin girls showing continuing growth discrepancy at 6 weeks. Twin 1 (right) birth weight 3.18 kg. Twin 2 (left): 1.55 kg.

Intrapair Discordance in Growth

Discrepancies in birth weight are commoner and larger within MZ pairs. This is mainly due to the cases of fetofetal transfusion syndrome when the haemodynamic imbalance results in transfer of nutrition from donor to recipient (see p.46). Another cause of unequal fetal growth in monochorionic twins is eccentric insertion of one of the two umbilical cords into the placental disc. One twin fetus may then receive less of the available maternal nutrition than its co-twin (Figs. 4.3 and 4.4).

Dichorionic twins, although less often, can be grossly discordant in size. This is more common when the placentae are separate than when they are fused (Fujikura and Froehlich 1971).

When a single umbilical artery is found in twins it is more commonly the smaller twin that is affected. Whether the absence of an artery, by reducing fetomaternal circulation, is responsible for the poor fetal growth or whether some other detrimental factor disturbs both growth and umbilical artery development is unknown.

Monitoring Fetal Growth

The monitoring of fetal development by ultrasound scan has given us a new insight into the growth of the living fetus. Before ultrasound was introduced studies had necessarily been limited to dead or prematurely delivered fetuses which were to some degree abnormal.

There have now been a number of studies on fetal biparietal diameters (BPD) in twin pregnancy (Divers and Hemsell 1979; Leveno et al. 1979, Fig. 4.5). Schneider (1978) found that the 50th centile for twins is nearer the tenth centile for singletons. However, Crane et al. (1980) showed that if discordant twins (those whose birth weight differed by over 25%) were excluded then BPD of twins were the same as those of appropriately grown singletons. In

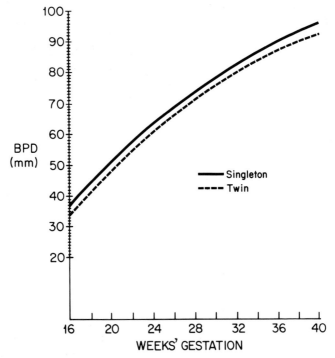

Fig. 4.5. Mean twin and singleton biparietal diameters between 16 and 40 weeks' gestation. From Leveno et al. (1979) by permission of the author and the editors of the *American Journal of Obstetrics and Gynecology.*

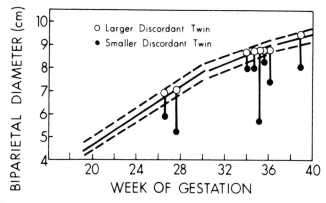

Fig. 4.6. Biparietal diameters in eight pairs of discordant-weight twins plotted against the normal range for singletons. The measurements were the last taken before delivery. From Crane et al. 1980. Reprinted with permission from The American College of Obstetricians and Gynecologists.

discordant pairs the BPD of the heavier twin was similar to that of both concordant twins and of singletons, whereas the lighter twin had, in many cases, a BPD well below the normal range (Fig. 4.6).

Discordance in BPD which can be detected during the second trimester is most likely to be due to the fetofetal transfusion syndrome and carries a high mortality. Diverging BPD after the 30th week, however, has a better prognosis and is probably a reflection of unequal maternofetal transfer to the two fetuses (Crane et al. 1980).

Recently it has been suggested that other ultrasound measurements may give more reliable indications of fetal growth. Neilson (1982) found that the product of the crown–rump length and the trunk area identified all growth-retarded twin fetuses whereas, in an earlier study, 44% had been missed on BPD measurements.

Alphafetoprotein

Maternal serum AFP levels may also give some indication of fetal wellbeing.

As with singletons (Wald et al. 1977), a negative correlation has been shown between mean birth weight of a twin pair and maternal AFP levels measured between the 11th and 24th weeks (Wald et al. 1978). Wald et al. (1979) offered this as an explanation for their later finding of higher AFP levels in MZ than DZ twin pregnancies. MZ twins are on average lighter than DZ.

However, Brock et al. (1979) suggested that the results could predict two separate groups of low-birth-weight twins. He found that high AFP levels were associated with preterm delivery whereas a low AFP provided a warning of early intrauterine growth retardation.

THE EFFECTS OF A SHARED BLOOD CIRCULATION

One in four pairs of twins have an additional influence on their intrauterine development and that is the effect of a shared circulation (see p. 77). In many instances monochorionic twins harmoniously share a 'third circulation' without apparent ill-effect. Occasionally, as in the case of acardia, the fetus is actually dependent on this intrapair circulation for survival. In other instances, as in the fetofetal transfusion syndrome, the results may be disastrous.

The Chronic Fetofetal Transfusion Syndrome

The chronic fetofetal transfusion syndrome is the result of an intrauterine blood transfusion between a pair of monochorionic twins. It is the cause of some of the greatest disturbances in twin fetal development. Not only may unequal growth occur but the effects of anaemia and polycythaemia may be so profound as to cause death to one or both fetuses.

It is a commoner condition than generally realized. Rausen et al. (1965) found evidence of this syndrome in 19 of 130 (15%) monochorionic twin pregnancies. They felt that even this figure was an underestimation of the true incidence.

The severe growth retardation frequently seen in the donor twin shows that the transfusion is a chronic process often lasting many weeks (Fig. 4.7). Indeed the syndrome has been recognized as early as the 10th week of pregnancy in a pair of aborted twin fetuses (Benirschke 1972).

The donor twin is commonly smaller—invariably so when there are large intrapair weight discrepancies. [When the twins are of similar weight they are likely to be examples of the acute type of fetofetal transfusion syndrome (see p.65).] The poor growth of the donor is due to the loss of nutrients together with haemoglobin to the co-twin. There may also be reduced maternofetal transfer of

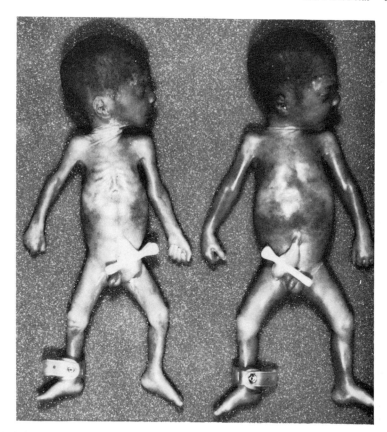

Fig. 4.7. Fetofetal transfusion syndrome in 24 weeks' gestation aborted twins. Donor (left) weight 670 g, Hb 11.8 g/100 ml; Recipient (right) weight 830 g, Hb 17.5 g/100 ml.

amino acids across the grossly abnormal and oedematous placenta (Bryan 1977a).

Differences in the weights of some of the fetal organs may be even greater than those of the body as a whole. Most information has been provided by Naeye (1963, 1964a,b, 1965; Naeye and Letts 1964), who found that all organs of the recipient were significantly larger than those of the donor and that the donor's were like those of singletons suffering from intrauterine malnutrition. The sparsity of lymphoid tissue in spleen and thymus is typical. Changes in the cardiovascular system were particularly striking. The cardiac mass of the recipient was sometimes twice that of the donor. Histologically there was hyperplasia of myocardial fibres and an increase in muscle mass in both systemic and pulmonary arteries. Renal glomeruli of the recipient were more mature not only than their donor's but also than singletons'. It is suggested that this acceleration in development occurs in response to the increased blood volume which, in turn, probably accounts for the high fetal urine production which may cause gross polyhydramnios. This increase in amniotic fluid is often the first clue to a disturbance in the fetofetal haemodynamic balance.

Chimerism

Occasionally a DZ twin has two distinct blood groups. He is then known as a chimera and must have received blast cells from his twin during intrauterine life. This condition can occur only in the rare situation of placental anastomoses in a fused (dichorionic) placenta (Nylander and Osunkoya 1970; Corney 1975*b*). Such twins are, at least partly, immunologically tolerant of each other and will, for instance, accept each other's skin grafts (Benirschke and Kim 1973).

CONGENITAL MALFORMATIONS

The study of congenital malformations in twins is beset with special problems. On the one hand it is difficult to collect a large enough sample if a random population is studied and, on the other, if the study is limited to malformed twins, there tends to be an over-representation of concordant pairs. Furthermore if one twin has died a malformed survivor may not be recognized as a twin (Carter 1965). It is probably for these reasons that figures for incidence and concordance vary greatly between studies (Benirschke and Kim 1973). The definitions of congenital malformations also vary from one study to another. This may invalidate comparisons between twin and singleton populations from different studies.

It is now generally accepted that congenital malformations are more common in twins than singletons (Dunn 1965; Hendricks 1966; Onyskowová et al. 1971), but that the increase is confined to like-sexed pairs (Stevenson et al. 1966; Hay and Wehrung 1970). More recent studies have shown that it is the MZ group which is responsible for the high incidence (Myrianthopoulos and Melnick 1977; Schinzel et al. 1979).

A number of major and multiple malformations, which are likely to be the result of an insult in early embryonic life, are over-represented amongst MZ twins whereas defects of later origin such as cleft palate and some types of congenital heart disease are as common in both types of twins (Schinzel et al. 1979).

Why MZ twins should have such a high incidence of malformations, particularly major ones, is not clear. Many authors favour the idea that MZ twinning is in itself a form of congenital malformation and that the unknown agent responsible for the twinning process (see p.15) may also cause the structural anomaly (Smith et al. 1976). In support of this theory is the fact that conjoined twins have a particularly high incidence of malformations (unrelated to their conjoined state) and they may even be discordant for these.

Other workers have suggested that the shared placental and fetal circulation of monochorionic twins provides a less favourable environment for fetal development (Bulmer 1970). However, studies by Melnick and Myrianthopoulos (1979) have failed to show a higher incidence of malformations amongst MZ twins with monochorionic placentation than with dichorionic. The same authors have offered another explanation. They suggest that the disruption of the developmental genetic clock of the embryo caused by the zygote division and the temporary reduction in cell number could cause a numerical and temporal biochemical disadvantage in the two 'new' embryos. This might make them more susceptible to the action of subtle environmental agents.

With the exception of neural tube defects there is a higher concordance for all malformations amongst MZ than DZ twins. For instance an MZ twin with cleft palate is at least five times more likely than a DZ to have an affected co-twin (Metrakos et al. 1958; Douglas 1958; Hay and Wehrung 1970).

Nevertheless MZ twins are still more likely than not to be discordant for most malformations. This suggests that environmental influences, as well as genetic determinants, play an important role for the majority of malformations. Even syndromes with multiple anomalies such as Klippel–Feil, Goldenhar, De Lange and Rubinstein–Taybi are often discordant (Schinzel et al. 1979).

No single malformation with invariable MZ concordance has been reported. The Prader–Willi syndrome is the one malformation complex in which all reported cases have been concordant. However, of a total of five cases at least one showed a marked intrapair variance in severity (Schinzel et al. 1979).

Congenital Heart Disease

A number of workers have found congenital heart disease to be more common in like-sexed twins than in singletons (McKeown and Record 1960; Hay and Wehrung 1970; Mitchell et al. 1971; Myrianthopoulos 1975; Layde et al. 1980).

MZ twins appear to account for this increase as Anderson (1977) found that 58% of twins in his study were MZ and similar trends have been reported by others (Campbell 1961; Kenna et al. 1975; Noonan 1978). Interestingly, however, the concordance rates amongst MZ twins are relatively low. Figures range from 6.8% to 46% (Campbell 1961; Nora et al. 1967; Jorgensen et al. 1971; Anderson 1977). The reason why only one of MZ twins is commonly affected is not clear but haemodynamic differences in early fetal life could affect the development of the cardiovascular system.

Positional Defects

All twins would be likely to suffer from positional defects due to the intrauterine congestion and relative restriction of movement. Minor foot deformities and skull asymmetry may be more common in twins (Schinzel et al. 1979) but usually resolve quickly and spontaneously. They are rarely mentioned in twin studies. True talipes equino varus and congenital dislocation of the hip appear to have a strong genetic component (Idelberger 1929, 1951).

Chromosomal Anomalies

Most known chromosomal anomalies have been reported in twins (Benirschke and Kim 1973). These are usually discordant in DZ twins and, surprisingly, also occasionally in MZ (Riekhof et al. 1972; Scott and Ferguson-Smith 1973). The twins are then known as heterokaryotes. In these MZ cases it is assumed that the maldistribution of chromosomes occurred at about the same time as the twinning process (post-zygotic non-disjunction).

Heterokaryotes XY/XO are the explanation for the occasional pair of MZ twins of different sexes. Indeed discordance is common in Turner's syndrome (Riekhof et al. 1972).

Klinefelter's syndrome (XXY) appears to be commoner than expected not only in twins but also in their relatives (Hoefnagel and Benirschke 1962; Nielsen 1966). The reason for this is not known. Hoefnagel suggests that there may be a relationship between the chromosomal error and the twinning process.

Down's Syndrome (mongolism)

Unlike other congenital malformations trisomy 21 is not increased in twins. Indeed the incidence is actually lower in MZ twins than in singletons (Keay 1958; MacDonald 1964; Hay and Wehrung 1970). It has been suggested that this low incidence may be due to a higher early loss of affected MZ embryos due to the combined insult of zygote cleavage and chromosomal imbalance.

Rare cases of MZ twins discordant for trisomy 21 have been reported (Scott and Ferguson-Smith 1973) and in these the abnormality must have occurred after fertilization.

Not surprisingly concordance in DZ twins is unusual as two separate chromosomal anomalies would be necessary. Nevertheless several authors have reported a somewhat higher incidence than would be expected even allowing for maternal age (MacDonald 1964; Bulmer 1970). This suggests that some women may have a predisposition to the chromosomal anomaly.

Neural Tube Defects

The association of neural tube defects with twinning is complex and still ill understood. Reports vary as to the incidence of these malformations in twins but anencephaly, at least, appears to be more common in MZ twins than singletons (Hay and Wehrung 1970).

In view of the known familial incidence of neural tube defects it might be expected that concordance in MZ twins would be high. The reverse is in fact true. Concordance is rare and no higher amongst MZ than DZ twins (Carter 1965). The explanation for this may be that it is the very inequality in blood circulation through the placental anastomoses that is responsible for the defect.

Another aspect of the relationship between neural tube defects and twinning has been explored by Knox (1970, 1974). In his epidemiological study of neural tube defects he showed that there is a general association between the incidence of anencephaly and dizygotic twinning rates. He suggests that neural tube defects could arise as a result of interaction between two fetuses. Maternal tissues might accept less easily two antigenically different and competing trophoblasts. When the two trophoblasts made contact this might lead to an interaction where one fetus was destroyed and the other left with a neural tube defect.

Further support for the idea of an association between twinning and neural tube defects has been provided by Le Marec et al. (1978). They found a significantly higher incidence of twins amongst the parents of 155 children with neural tube defects.

Acardia

This, the most severe of all malformations, occurs in about one in 30 000 deliveries (Benirschke and Kim 1973). It must be confined to multiple pregnancy as survival of the fetus is dependent on a shared circulation with the (usually normal) co-twin. There is some suggestion that acardia may occur more often in triplet pregnancies (Schinzel et al. 1979).

Acardiac fetuses vary from a mass of amorphous tissue to an incomplete but well-formed fetus weighing up to 3.5 kg. They are usually attached to a monochorionic placenta by an umbilical cord with only one artery.

An imbalance in the interfetal circulation resulting in atrophy of the heart has been held responsible for these acardiac monsters. However, this may not be the explanation in all cases as chromosomal abnormalities have been detected in some acardiac fetuses (Kerr and Rashad 1966; Scott and Ferguson-Smith 1973). This suggests that the cause may be more fundamental. Furthermore, specific abnormalities are not uncommon and in several cases the co-twin has anomalies of the same type. In a review of 85 cases the incidence of malformations in the co-twin was as high as 10% (Schinzel et al. 1979).

Fetus-in-fetu, which is considered to be an MZ twin, may well have a similar origin to acardiac twins (Janovski 1962; Grant and Pearn 1969) as may another form of twinning, the sacrococcygeal teratoma (Gross et al. 1951).

Conjoined Twins

This tragic malformation is a form of MZ twinning in which the division of the zygote is incomplete. The cause is unknown but assumed to be the same as for MZ twins in general (see p.15). The increased incidence of severe additional malformations in these cases suggests that the aetiological factors may be common to both MZ twinning and some malformations (Schinzel et al. 1979).

In view of its rarity it is not surprising to find that reports on the incidence of conjoined twinning vary. The figure given by Bulmer (1970) of one in 100 000 maternities is probably too low. Twice that incidence is more likely (Hanson 1975), that is, one in every 200 MZ twin maternities. There are no known predisposing factors although there have been occasional reports of geographical (Bhettay et al. 1975; Zake 1982) and seasonal (Milham 1966) clustering.

All studies have reported a low sex ratio. Indeed in Milham's (1966) study of 22 cases 20 were female. There has been only one report of a second set of conjoined twins in a family (Hamon and Dinno 1978) and, as would be expected with MZ twinning, a family history of twins is not particularly common. The occasional case of a conjoined pair with a normal triplet has been reported (Tan et al. 1971; Vestergaard 1972). In at least one case the normal fetus has had its own amniotic sac which suggests that zygote division must have taken place on two separate occasions (Vestergaard 1972).

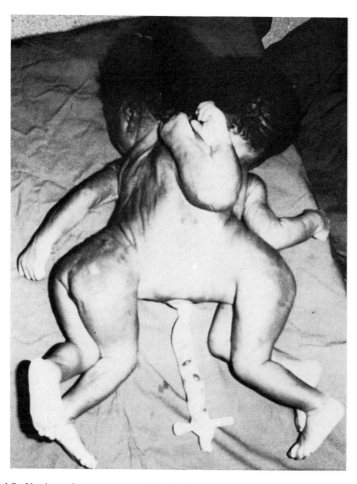

Fig. 4.8. Newborn thoracopagus conjoined twins.

A surprising finding in Milham's (1966) study was that of a high stillbirth rate in previous pregnancies. Seven of a total of 33 pregnancies had ended with the delivery of a stillborn infant which suggests that maternal factors may be of importance in the aetiology of conjoined twins (Milham 1966).

The site and extent of fusion of the fetuses is infinitely variable. Thoracopagus is the commonest form of fusion and accounts for over 70% of cases (Fig. 4.8). Pyopagus is the next commonest. The full range of conjoined twins is listed in Table 4.1 (Guttmacher and Nichols 1967).

Table 4.1. Types of conjoined twins

Inferior conjunction
Diprosopus—two faces with one head and body
Dicephalus—two heads and one body
Ischiopagus—inferior sacrococcygeal fusion
Pygopagus—posterolateral sacrococcygeal fusion

Superior conjunction
Dipygus—two pelves and four legs
Syncephalus—facial ± thoracic fusion
Craniopagus—cranial fusion

Mid conjunction
Thoracopagus—thoracic fusion
Omphalopagus—fusion from umbilicus to xiphoid cartilage
Rachipagus—vertebral fusion above sacrum

The feasibility of separating conjoined twins obviously depends on the site and extent of fusion and the degree to which organs are shared, as well as the availability of appropriate surgical expertise. Unfortunately the diagnosis of conjoined twins is too often made after the onset of labour. Thus the mother is not able to have an elective caesarean section which would reduce the risk of damage to herself and the babies. Nor is she likely to be in a hospital equipped to deal with such a rare and complicated case. Suspicion of conjoined twins should be aroused in all cases of polyhydramnios in multiple pregnancies and also in those where an x-ray reveals an abnormal fetal posture (Rudolph et al. 1967).

Nowadays many conjoined twins can be successfully separated and several detailed descriptions are given in the comprehensive review of conjoined twins edited by Bergsma (1967). In the same volume Pepper (1967) considers the ethical dilemma that conjoined twins present. First in considering initial resuscitation of the infants at birth, then of surgical separation, particularly if the survival of one is likely to be at the expense of the other. Finally he discusses the long term psychological adjustment of those who have been separated as well as those who remain fused.

A number of conjoined twins have lived surprisingly full and active lives (Gedda 1961). Some—both men and women—have married and had children. Many have shown different tastes and temperaments which at times have led to intrapair tensions. Perhaps it is more surprising that others have managed to live together in harmony.

Many physiological responses of a conjoined pair may be autonomous. Heart rhythms may differ and change independently in response to external stimuli. If one of a pair becomes pregnant the other may continue to menstruate.

The xiphopags pair, Chang and Eng (1811–74) were the original 'Siamese twins'. They married two sisters and one had 12 children and the other ten.

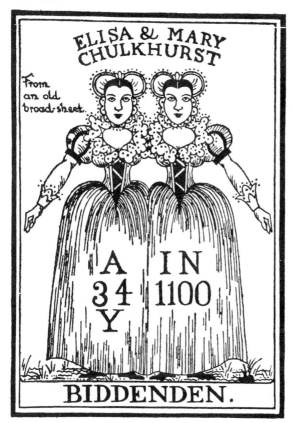

Fig. 4.9. The Chulkhurst sisters. Conjoined twins.

One of the earliest and most famous English pairs were Elisa and Mary Chulkhurst from Kent who are depicted on the village sign as 'The Biddenden Maids' (Fig. 4.9). Born in 1100, they were laterally joined in the scapular and gluteal regions. After their death at the age of 34 the Chulkhurst Charity was established. Part of this includes the distribution of biscuits embossed with their figures each Easter.

In all cases of unseparated twins the death of one is quickly followed by the death of the other even if there is no structural cause for this. It is likely that thromboplastin from the dead twin crosses into the survivor's circulation and causes disseminated intravascular coagulation.

In both the 'Siamese' and the Chulkhurst pairs one twin died a few hours before the other. On both occasions the survivor chose to die rather than accept surgical separation.

INTRAUTERINE INFECTIONS

Intrauterine infections commonly affect both twins but occasionally one twin alone suffers the teratogenic insult (Penrose 1937; Forrester et al. 1966; Satge et al. 1966; Henriksen et al. 1968; Shearer et al. 1972). However, in at least one of the cases reported it was shown that the other twin had in fact been infected but suffered no lasting damage (Forrester et al. 1966). It may be that these two fetuses were infected at a slightly, but critically, different stage in their embryological development (see below).

Such discordance has only once been reported in MZ twins (Penrose 1937) and this case must be interpreted with caution as comprehensive tests of zygosity were not included. Discordance in MZ twins could presumably only occur in those with dichorionic placentation.

Later in pregnancy the presenting twin could, theoretically, be at greater risk of infection from organisms in the genital tract. Benirschke and Driscoll (1967) found that chorioamnionitis was invariably associated with the first twin when only one sac was involved. However, there have been no reports of an increased incidence of such infections in firstborn twins. Nevertheless the finding of higher levels of the fetally synthesized immunoglobulins M and A in firstborn twins does suggest that the ascending organisms may have provided antigenic stimulation for the synthesis of these immunoglobulins (Bryan 1976).

TERATOGENIC EFFECTS OF DRUGS

As with infections it appears that there may be intrapair differences in susceptibility to the teratogenic effects of drugs, including alcohol. One twin may be severely affected whereas the other may have only minor or no signs at all (Mellin and Katzenstein 1962; Lenz 1966; Loughnan et al. 1973; Christoffel and Salafsky 1975; Schmidt and Salzano 1980). Lenz (1966) suggested that, at least in the case of thalidomide, the teratogenic effect of which is sharply limited, this occasional discordance in a pair of twins could be due to the insult acting at the very beginning or end of the sensitive period. One DZ twin may thus be a few days retarded or accelerated in development and therefore escape unharmed.

RHESUS ISOIMMUNIZATION AND HYDROPS FETALIS IN TWINS

Rhesus isoimmunization occurs in twins as in singletons. Management, however, is often much more complicated. Not only is it technically more difficult to perform amniocentesis and intrauterine blood transfusions in multiple pregnancy but decisions on management may be far more difficult. The life of one fetus may have to be sacrificed or at least risked for the sake of the healthy survival of the other (Nylander and MacGillivray 1975*b*). The risk of an intrauterine death of the more severely affected fetus if the pregnancy is allowed to continue often has to be weighed against the chances of losing both infants from the complications of prematurity if the babies are delivered too early. Selective intrauterine transfusion is possible only in skilled hands.

With dizygotic twins one only may be affected (Beischer et al. 1969). Even if both are rhesus sensitized the degree may differ according to their ABO blood grouping. Fetuses with the same ABO blood group as their mother's tend to be more severely affected than those with different ones. There are instances where severe oedema (hydrops fetalis) has occurred in only one of MZ rhesus-immunized twins (Kloosterman 1963; Fig. 4.10). Here genetic differences cannot be responsible and differences in placental function becomes the most likely explanation. Differences in the placental transfer of the maternally derived immunoglobulin G, fetal plasma levels of albumin and colloid osmotic pressure may all be of importance (Barnes et al. 1977).

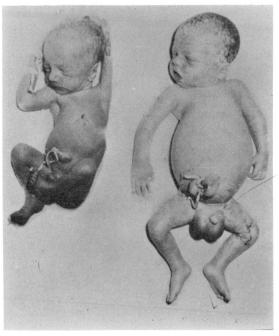

Fig. 4.10. Monozygotic twins with severe rhesus isoimmunization. The smaller baby survived after two exchange transfusions while the hydropic one died after 15 minutes. From Kloosterman (1963) by permission of the author.

Among the vast array of causes of hydrops fetalis there are a number specific to multiple pregnancy. Either or both twins in the fetofetal transfusion syndrome may become hydropic (Hibbard 1959; Macafee et al. 1970)—the recipient, as a result of cardiac failure due to hypervolaemia and increased blood viscosity. The donor may become hydropic as a result of anaemia and hypoalbuminaemia but surprisingly this is less common.

The abnormal circulation of an acardiac twin may cause oedema and the co-twin may also become oedematous due to cardiac failure from the increased load of a second fetal circulation.

INTRAUTERINE DEATH

Fetus Papyraceus

It is not uncommon to find the remains of a fetus compressed and embedded in the placenta of a healthy single baby (Benirschke and Driscoll 1967; Fig. 4.11). This fetus is known as a fetus papyraceus and the mother is usually unaware that she ever had a twin pregnancy. Most of these fetuses are the result of death in the second trimester. Earlier in the pregnancy a dead fetus is usually reabsorbed whereas the fetus that dies in the third trimester becomes macerated but not compressed.

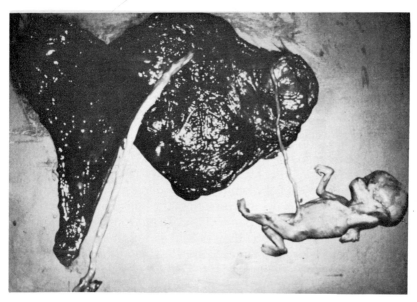

Fig. 4.11. Fetus papyraceus attached to a twin placenta. The twin was normal. By permission of H.G. Kohler.

The fetofetal transfusion syndrome and knotting of umbilical cords in monoamniotic twins account for the deaths of some of these fetuses. However a large number of fetus papyraceus are dichorionic twins (Kindred 1944) so other explanations such as separation of the placenta or blood group incompatibility must be sought in these cases.

Disseminated Intravascular Coagulation

Most twins survive the intrauterine death of their co-twin physically, at least, unharmed. However, in monochorionic twins, who share a placental blood circulation, the survivor may have severe problems from disseminated intravascular coagulation. Thromboplastin from the macerated fetus transfers to the live twin and causes intravascular coagulation with all its complications such as haemorrhage, anaemia and jaundice. Clots and debris from the dead fetus form emboli which may cause ischaemia and necrosis to organs, particularly the brain and kidney (Reisman and Pathak 1966; Moore et al. 1969; Koranyi and Kovacs 1975; Durkin et al. 1976; Melnick 1977; Yoshioka et al. 1979).

If one fetus dies early in pregnancy emboli may disrupt the development of the survivor. Schinzel et al. (1979) suggest that some congenital deformities such as aplasia cutis, hydranencephaly, porencephaly and intestinal atresia may sometimes result from such ischaemic insults in a twin pregnancy. In a study of 113 cases of aplasia cutis Mannino et al. (1977) found that as many as 15 had an MZ fetus papyraceus twin.

Later Intrauterine Death

About twice as many twins are stillborn as singletons. There are several reasons for this high fetal mortality. The maternal supply line is more likely to fail when two fetuses have to be sustained. One fetus often receives more nutrition than the other, but monitoring of individual fetal welfare, particularly if ultrasound scans are not available, may be difficult. Signs of fetal distress may be missed and the opportunity for active intervention lost. In other cases the life of one fetus may be deliberately risked if an induced premature delivery would jeopardize the chances of survival for the other (healthier) twin. This situation may arise in cases of blood group incompatibility. Finally there are the added hazards, peculiar to twins, of interfetal vascular disturbances such as the fetofetal transfusion syndrome.

5. Twin Delivery

The delivery of twins has added hazards not only because of the likelihood of prematurity but also because the fetal presentation is more likely to be abnormal. For these reasons a twin delivery should whenever possible take place where full consultant obstetric, paediatric and anaesthetic staff are available.

PARENTAL ANXIETIES

Parents are usually aware of the real risks. They may also have unnecessary fears and misconceptions and it is important that these should be recognized and allayed where possible. It is particularly important for those who have only recently realized that they are having twins and have had little time to gain information.

Many mothers fear a longer and more painful labour. Indeed some have started labour in the belief that they must go through the whole process twice over. In fact, there is no evidence that labour is prolonged in multiple pregnancy (see p.63). It is often more uncomfortable due to abdominal distension but the contractions themselves are no more painful. Parents are anxious too about the outcome for their babies and this anxiety may be reinforced by the number of medical personnel that gather as the time for delivery approaches. The mother may well think that something serious is afoot to require such medical manpower. It is important that she be briefed beforehand that many are there to watch and learn and she should have the option of reducing the audience should she so wish. Few mothers do.

As paediatric staff should always be involved with a twin delivery it is helpful if the paediatrician can meet the mother during the antenatal period or, at least, during the early stages of labour. She may well welcome the opportunity to ask questions at this time.

LABOUR

Onset

The greater the number of fetuses, the earlier is the labour likely to start. Many studies have shown that the average length of gestation for twin pregnancies is approximately 260 days (McKeown and Record 1952; Karn and Penrose 1952; Guttmacher and Kohl 1958; Butler and Alberman 1969; Stucki et al. 1982) compared with 280 days for singletons. The incidence of preterm delivery (less than 37 weeks' gestation) is between 20 and 30% (Butler and Alberman 1969; Kaupilla et al. 1975) and is higher amongst primigravidae (Kaupilla et al. 1975; Khoo and Green 1975; Weekes et al. 1977c) and younger mothers (Weekes et al. 1977c).

What causes the onset of labour is uncertain. Uterine overdistension can be at most a contributory factor. Redford (1982) found, in his ultrasound study of uterine growth in twin pregnancy, that there was no relation between uterine distension and onset of preterm labour. Indeed preterm delivery was more often preceded by impaired than accelerated uterine growth. Were uterine distension alone responsible, labour would start much sooner, that is, at the time when the combined weight of the fetuses was that of the average-term singleton.

The increase in circulating hormones of the fetal pituitary/ adrenal system in a multiple pregnancy may well affect the timing of labour. Effacement of the cervix may also play a part in the early onset of labour. In a multiple pregnancy the cervix may be prematurely effaced, possibly due to the increased pressure from the presenting fetus.

As prematurity is the single most important cause of the high perinatal mortality in twin pregnancies, prevention of an early onset of labour is of paramount importance. Unfortunately attempts to do this with twin pregnancies have, so far, been relatively unsuccessful. Most maternity units recommend bed rest for several weeks from the 30th week, particularly for primigravidae, for whom the risks are high and for whom a stay in hospital is less disruptive to family life. Results conflict and there has as yet been no convincing evidence of a beneficial effect (Editorial 1977).

Oral doses of β-sympathomimetic drugs over several weeks have also been tried but results have, so far, been disappointing; (O'Connor et al. 1979; MacGillivray 1982). In view of the premature cervical dilatation in many multiple pregnancies cervical suturing could theoretically be of benefit but this has not yet been demonstrated either (Weekes et al. 1977*b*). Indeed some workers consider it to be contraindicated (Sinha et al. 1979).

Until more is known of the pathogenesis of preterm labour in multiple pregnancy the main means of reducing the perinatal mortality must be to ensure that the diagnosis is made early and that facilities for intensive care of the babies are available.

Duration of Labour

The relative duration of labour in single and multiple pregnancies can no longer be validly assessed as in current obstetric practice slow labour is often accelerated. However, in earlier studies it was found, perhaps surprisingly, that labour was no longer in multiple than in single pregnancies (Bender 1952; Danielson 1960; Garrett 1960). In addition Garrett (1960) found that the proportion of labours that were prolonged beyond 36 hours was no greater. Eastman (1961) suggested that this was due to pre-labour cervical dilatation resulting in a shorter latent phase. Thus, despite the longer active phase needed to overcome the relative uterine inertia caused by overdistension, the total length of labour was not increased. Friedman and Sachtleben's (1964) findings in 184 twin pregnancies later confirmed Eastman's theory.

Although labour is not prolonged and contractions not necessarily any more painful the mother of twins is often distressed. Her general discomfort may be quite severe due to the distension and weight of the uterus. Her distress is often increased by her justifiably greater level of anxiety.

Presentation

Up to one-third of twin infants present by the breech (Portes and Granjon 1946; Guttmacher and Kohl 1958)—with all the well-known risks that go with this—in contrast to 3.5% of singletons. Kaupilla et al. (1975) found that the perinatal mortality was twice as high in breech- as in vertex-delivered twins.

In only 40–45% of cases do both babies present in the most favourable way, by the vertex (Portes and Granjon 1946; Potter and Fuller 1949; Guttmacher and Kohl 1958; Zuckerman and Brzezinski 1961; Farooqui et al. 1973). In 30–40% of cases one will be vertex and one breech (Portes and Granjon 1946; Guttmacher and Kohl 1958; Farooqui et al. 1973) and in this group the vertex-presenting twin is born first in three out of four instances (Portes and Granjon 1946).

One baby may have a transverse lie and the other vertex (5%) or breech (1.5%). Very occasionally both may have a transverse lie. These less favourable forms of presentation inevitably lead to an increased incidence of instrumental deliveries and caesarean sections—the incidence varying according to the practice of different centres.

COMPLICATIONS OF DELIVERY

In addition to the complications of malpresentation there are a number of hazards peculiar to a twin delivery.

Locking

Because of the catastrophic effect of this complication of twin delivery obstetric textbooks tend to devote a disproportionate amount of space to the locking of twins. The impression gained is that it is not uncommon. In fact it is extremely rare—in the order of one in 1000 twin deliveries.

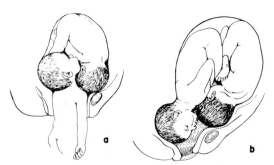

Fig. 5.1. Locking of twins. (a) Chin-to-chin. (b) Collision of two heads. From MacGillivray (1975*b*) by permission of the author and W.B. Saunders. Co. Ltd.

Nissen (1958) reviewed the literature up to 1957 and found 69 cases and another 50 or so have been reported since (Adams and Fetterhoff 1971; Khunda 1972). He divided the cases into four groups according to the different means of locking (Fig. 5.1). The first is 'collision', where contact of fetal parts between the twins prevents engagement of either. The second is 'impaction', where the impaction of fetal parts of one twin into the body of the other forces partial engagement of both together. The third is 'compaction', where the presenting parts of both fetuses become fully engaged in the pelvis and prevent further descent. The fourth, 'interlocking', is where the underside of both chins are in such close apposition as to prevent delivery of the firstborn breech.

The cause of locking is unknown but has been variously ascribed to the small size of the fetuses in relation to the mother's pelvis, to oligo-hydramnios and premature rupture of the amniotic membranes, to hypertonicity of the uterus and to the use of oxytocins. All of these may be contributory factors. The condition is much more common in primigravidae (Nissen 1958; Khunda 1972) and may occasionally be associated with uterine abnormalities (Parmar and Mulgund 1968; Theron 1969). It is probably more common in monoamniotic pregnancies as Nissen (1958) found seven cases in his series of a total of 69 pairs of locked twins.

Unfortunately, locking is rarely appreciated until part of the presenting fetus has already delivered. This makes vaginal disentanglement extremely difficult. Even with caesarean section the mortality rate is high—43% in Nissen's (1958) series and 31% in Khunda's (1972). Both authors found that the risk was much higher to the leading baby.

The Acute Fetofetal Transfusion Syndrome

In contrast to the more generally recognized chronic fetofetal transfusion syndrome (see p.46) this condition, also confined to monochorionic twins, actually occurs during labour. As a result of a haemodynamic imbalance in the fetoplacentofetal unit blood is transfused from one fetus (the donor) to the other (the recipient). Presumably this is due to changes in intravascular pressures across the large-vessel anastomoses (see p.77) secondary to the changing uterine pressures of labour. One fetus becomes acutely hypervolaemic and later polycythaemic and the other hypovolaemic and then anaemic. Both may die of cardiac failure if not treated immediately (see p.95).

Exsanguination of the Second Twin

As the great majority, if not all, of monochorionic placentae have vascular communications between the two sets of umbilical vessels haemorrhage from the unclamped placental end of the umbilical cord of the first twin can cause severe blood loss to the second. It is now general practice to ligate both ends of the cord so this complication should no longer occur.

Vasa Praevia

Whitehouse and Kohler (1960) reported six cases of vasa praevia (when blood vessels traverse the placental membranes in front of the presenting fetal part) in multiple pregnancy. All were associated with monochorionic placentae and, thus, rupture of the vessels could exsanguinate not only the first but both babies.

As a velamentous insertion is much commoner in twin pregnancies (Benirschke and Driscoll 1967) it is likely that vasa praevia also occurs more frequently.

Monoamniotic Twins

A few MZ twins share an amniotic sac and as a result their intrauterine life is particularly hazardous. Monoamniotic twins are thought to result from the later splitting of the developing zygote when the amniotic membrane has already developed. It is possible, however, that some cases are due to the disintegration of an amniotic septum. A monoamniotic pair within a triplet pregnancy may also occur (Wharton et al. 1968).

Earlier authors reported an incidence of single amnions in twin pregnancies of less than 1% (Quigley 1935; Potter 1963) but more recent studies suggest that these were underestimations. Incidences of between 1 and 3% are now more common (Wharton et al. 1968; Fujikura and Froehlich 1971; Corney et al. 1972).

Females are much more common in monoamniotic pregnancies than in twins in general. James (1977) suggests that this may be because the sex of the zygote is associated with the time within the menstrual cycle that it is formed.

The main hazard to a monoamniotic fetus is entanglement of the umbilical cords (Fig. 5.2). Foglmann (1976) found that this occurred in 60% of over 200 cases of monoamniotic twins. This may lead to umbilical vessel occlusion with a high risk of anoxic

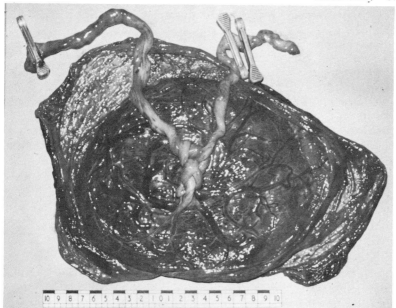

Fig. 5.2. Placenta of monoamniotic twins showing knotting of umbilical cords. By permission of Dr. J. Pryse-Davies.

death for both fetuses. Occasionally the cord of one twin may become tightly entwined around the neck of the other (Tagawa 1974). As the first twin is delivered it may not immediately be appreciated that the cord around its neck is that of the twin rather than its own.

Inevitably the incidence of knotting and indeed of death in these twins is likely to be overestimated as healthy twins with no cord entanglement may not be noticed to be monoamniotic. Certainly early reports give extremely high mortality rates. In reviewing 109 cases in 1935 Quigley found a 68% mortality rate and in only 17 pairs did both babies survive. More recent studies have shown a perinatal mortality rate between 30% and 50% (Benirschke and Driscoll 1967; Wharton et al. 1968; Tagawa 1974).

Unless amniography has had to be performed for other reasons (which is unlikely) the diagnosis of monoamniotic twins is rarely made until after the birth of the first twin. The absence of an amniotic membrane may then be noticed or, less commonly, a knotted cord may be apparent on the first twin (Goplerud 1964). The number of unsuspected monoamniotic twins will be greatly reduced when membrane relationships can be accurately determined by ultrasound scanning. Promising preliminary results on echography of the amniotic membranes have been reported from France (Bessis and Papiernick 1981).

THE UNDIAGNOSED TWIN

An unexpected second baby presents real problems, especially for medical staff who may be inexperienced and also ill-prepared for the complications of a twin delivery. The problem to the mother (and father) however, may be no smaller. At the height of her exhaustion and stress she has to cope with the shock and sudden need to relate to a second baby.

Although undiagnosed twins are less common now (see p.27) there are still many centres where it is expected that at least 15% of twin pregnancies will not be detected prior to birth.

The main dangers to the undiagnosed twin are those of a precipitate delivery before its presence has been realized or, more commonly, retention and fetal anoxia due to contraction of the uterus following administration of ergometrine.

BIRTH INTERVAL

It is now generally agreed that the hazards to the second fetus of a delay in delivery beyond 30 minutes outweigh any risks of active intervention. Most obstetricians prefer to see the second twin delivered within 20 minutes. Many consider the optimal time to be between 10 and 20 minutes (Spurway 1962; Benirschke and Kim 1973; Farr 1975) and believe that greater haste is harmful and associated with a significantly higher perinatal mortality rate (Farrell 1964). Others, however, feel the sooner the better (Corston 1957; Muller-Holve et al. 1976) and would recommend rupturing the second amniotic sac immediately after delivery of the first baby in order to prevent the cervix contracting again. On the other hand the advent of reliable monitoring of fetal wellbeing in labour may well alter obstetric practice in the future. Some obstetricians now consider that active intervention should only be undertaken if there are signs of fetal distress; that the actual duration of birth interval does not matter.

In the past the interval between the two deliveries was often several hours and occasionally much longer. The longest on record was that reported by Drucker et al. (1960) where the mother was delivered of a 375-g fetus and 65 days later of a 1390-g female infant. Unlike some other cases of prolonged intervals in which the mother had uteri didelphys (Williams and Cummings 1953; Dorgan and Clarke 1956; Green et al. 1961) her uterus was normal. A similar case was reported by Abrams (1957).

Intervals of more than an hour or so are now rare except in developing countries. Reports from some of these areas have confirmed the greatly increased risk run by the fetus which is retained. Adeleye (1972) studied 106 second twins in Nigeria who were retained for over 30 minutes. Many of the firstborn twins had been born outside the hospital. Retention was thought to be due to malpresentation in about half of the cases and to uterine inertia in the remainder. The perinatal mortality in the second twin was three times that of the first and, more significantly, rose to tenfold (47%) in those retained for over 2 hours.

There are exceptional circumstances when the interval is therapeutically prolonged for several weeks to allow the second fetus to mature. Thomsen (1978) describes a case in which the first baby was delivered at 27 weeks' gestation weighing 680 g. Labour-inhibiting drugs were then given and a cervical cerclage inserted. Labour did not recur for another 4 weeks, at which time a 1192-g infant was delivered, and survived. There were two separate placentae but both were retained until after the birth of the second baby. Infection was not a problem.

ANAESTHESIA

No medical team prepared for the delivery of twins is complete without an experienced anaesthetist. General anaesthesia as well as epidural analgesia are frequently required and sometimes, in the case of the second twin, at short notice.

With the greater discomfort of a twin labour nearly all mothers will require some form of analgesia. Those that cause respiratory depression, such as pethidine, should be avoided for the sake, particularly, of the second twin who is already likely to be embarrassed by reduced levels of oxygen.

Epidural analgesia is now the analgesic and anaesthetic of choice for twin deliveries. It has, amongst other things, the advantage that the mother is already prepared for any manoevres such as an internal version or instrumental delivery, that may be necessary for the second twin. The delay caused by preparation and induction of a general anaesthetic is avoided and, not least, the mother can still have the pleasure of seeing her baby as it is born.

Several workers have found that with epidural analgesia the metabolic balance of both babies compares favourably with other forms of analgesia (James et al. 1977; Jaschevatzky et al. 1977; Weekes et al. 1977a). Likewise neither the length of labour nor the incidence of instrumental deliveries was increased when epidural analgesia was used (Weekes et al. 1977a). Crawford (1975) actually found the delivery interval to be shorter in those mothers with this form of analgesia.

Maternal hypotension due to aorto-caval compression is a real danger and can lead to severe oxygen deprivation to both babies. Precautions must be taken to avoid this.

RISKS TO FIRST AND SECOND TWIN

Almost all recent studies show a higher perinatal mortality rate for the second-born twin than the first. Although many individual studies are inconclusive in that the difference between the two babies is not statistically significant, when analysed cumulatively the evidence is overwhelmingly in favour of the firstborn. In reviewing the literature on over 23 000 infants Wyshak and White (1963) found a perinatal mortality rate of 57.1 per 1000 for firstborn and 74.6 for second. In the 28 studies they analysed only two showed the reverse trend.

If one twin dies in utero the live one is generally delivered first. Even if macerated stillbirths are excluded from the figures, however, the loss of the second twin is still higher than that of the first (Guttmacher and Kohl 1958; Potter 1963; Koivisto et al. 1975).

In good obstetric units, where delay in the delivery of the second twin is avoided, the difference in the fate of the two infants is now becoming steadily less.

The leading twin has to dilate the cervix, and is therefore at greater risk, particularly if premature, than the second of intracranial haemorrhage from birth injury (Griffiths 1967). Theoretically the risk of infection ascending from the genital tract is also greater but there is scant evidence to support this (see p.56).

Weighted against the second twin is the risk of fetal anoxia particularly when delivery is delayed (Adeleye 1972) or when the second twin is undiagnosed; it is then in danger of being trapped in utero or conversely catapulted out with undue speed if oxytocin is given. The greater likelihood of malpresentation or a breech delivery requiring instrumental intervention add further hazards. The respiratory distress syndrome may occur in the second twin only or, if both are affected, the second twin is usually more severely affected and more likely to succumb (see p.89).

6. The Twin Placenta

Placentation may have a profound effect on the long-term development of twins. Yet all too often details are carelessly recorded and the value of many twin studies is greatly reduced by lack of information on this vital factor.

TYPES OF PLACENTA

There are three types of placenta—single, fused and separate. The site of implantation in the uterus, the zygosity and, in MZ twins, the timing of zygote division together determine the type found in a particular pregnancy. As DZ twins arise from two zygotes they always have individual placentae. Depending on their site of implantation these may remain entirely discrete or, if close, will fuse together partially, or completely, to form an apparently single placental disc. The relative frequency of these two types of dichorionic placentation cannot be determined satisfactorily from the literature; the criterion for fusion varies in different studies from a loose membranous attachment to firm adherence of placental tissues.

The type of placenta found in MZ twinning gives a good indication of the stage of development at which the zygote divided (Fig. 6.1). If division occurs during the first 3 days after fertilization the twins will have individual placentae.

Several workers (Potter 1963; Nylander 1970*b*; Fujikura and Froehlich 1971), although not all (Corney et al. 1972), have found that MZ dichorionic placentae are more likely to be fused than DZ

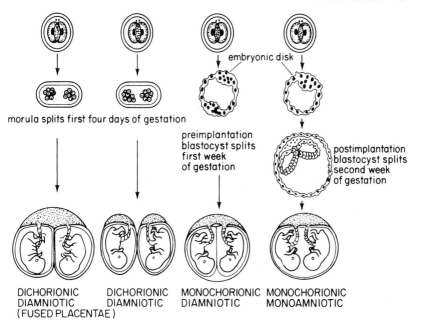

morula splits first four days of gestation

embryonic disk

preimplantation blastocyst splits first week of gestation

postimplantation blastocyst splits second week of gestation

DICHORIONIC DIAMNIOTIC (FUSED PLACENTAE)

DICHORIONIC DIAMNIOTIC

MONOCHORIONIC DIAMNIOTIC

MONOCHORIONIC MONOAMNIOTIC

Fig. 6.1. The development and placentation of monozygotic twins. From Fox (1978). By permission of the author and W.B. Saunders Co. Ltd.

(Corney 1975*b*). Fujikura and Froehlich (1971) suggest that this is due to an increased chance of adjacent implantation when the two zygotes come from the same fallopian tube which, of course, they always do in MZ twins.

There is probably no difference in function between fused and separate placentae per se but as placental function may be affected by the site of implantation it is not surprising that discrepancies in fetal growth in like-sexed DZ twins are greater in those with separate placentae (Fujikura and Froehlich 1971). If one placenta is sited on the posterior wall of the uterus and the other, for instance, near the cervix then the first will receive a greater uteroplacental blood flow and thus better nutrition for that fetus.

WEIGHT AND FUNCTION

At the same combined birth weight twins have heavier placentae than singletons and the discrepancy remains, although reduced, even when correction is made for differences in gestational age (McKeown and Record 1953; Gruenwald 1970) (Fig. 6.2).

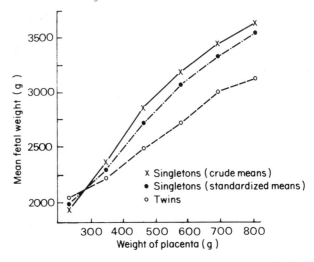

Fig. 6.2. Fetal weight in relation to placental weight in twins and singletons showing that for the same placental weight singletons are heavier than twins, even when standardized for gestational age. From McKeown and Record (1953) by permission of the authors and the editor of *Journal of Endocrinology.*

Little is known about placental function in multiple pregnancy. The relatively high placental:fetal ratio suggests that the function may well be reduced and that placental hypertrophy has been needed to compensate and sustain an adequate 'maternal supply line' to the fetus.

THE UMBILICAL CORD

Apart from some conjoined twins and the extremely rare case of monoamniotic twins with a forked cord, all twins have an individual umbilical cord. The cords may vary greatly in size and also in site of insertion into the placenta and both these factors may affect fetal nutrition (see Fig. 4.3). Abnormally inserted umbilical cords are more common in twin placentae (Benirschke and Driscoll 1967; Strong and Corney 1967) and intrapartum haemorrhage associated with a velamentous insertion contributes to the high perinatal mortality of multiple pregnancy.

The umbilical vessels, as in singletons, usually spiral in an anticlockwise direction but this is variable and Edmonds (1954) found that the direction may differ within a pair of twins.

Most workers have found that single umbilical arteries (SUA) are commoner in twins (Benirschke and Driscoll 1967; Strong and Corney 1967), although this was not confirmed by our own study (Bryan and Kohler 1974). Both the earlier studies found an incidence of over 3.5% in twins compared with under 1% in singletons (Bryan and Kohler 1974). As in singletons, malformations were more common in the twins with SUA but, apart from acardia, these malformations do not appear to be of a particular type. There is some indication that SUA is more common amongst MZ than DZ twins (Strong and Corney 1967; Boyd and Hamilton 1970) but the numbers are too small for a definite conclusion to be reached.

It is rare for twins to be concordant for SUA and, in general, the anomaly occurs in the smaller of the two infants (Seki and Strauss 1964; Kristofferson 1969; Bryan and Kohler 1974). This agrees with the finding of a higher incidence of SUA amongst small-for-dates singleton babies (Bryan and Kohler 1974).

PLACENTATION AND ZYGOSITY (Fig. 6.3.)

For many years it was believed that MZ and DZ twins could be distinguished by the number of chorionic membranes. Unfortunately this belief dies hard. It later became clear that some MZ twins must have dichorionic placentae; for by applying Weinberg's rule (1902) it was clear that more MZ twins should have existed than the number of twins found to have monochorionic placentae. This conclusion was supported by the observation that some twins with dichorionic placentae were physically indistinguishable. Later studies show that between 18.5 and 37.5% of MZ twins do in fact have placentae with two chorions (Corney 1975*b*).

In contrast it seems unlikely that human DZ twins ever have monochorionic placentae. In six studies none were found in a total of 3452 twin pairs of known zygosity (Corney 1975*b*). Occasional reports of monochorionic placentae in DZ pregnancies lack validity in that essential histological evidence is missing. Nylander and Osunkoya (1970) demonstrated the importance of this in their interesting case of unlike-sexed twins with an apparently monochorionic placenta. Only on histological investigation did they find fragments of chorionic tissue at the base of the septum from which they concluded that these must be remnants of a, now disintegrated, dichorionic septum.

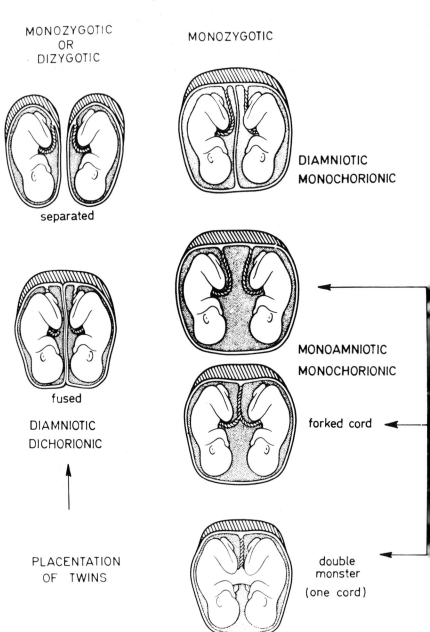

MONOZYGOTIC
OR
DIZYGOTIC

MONOZYGOTIC

separated

DIAMNIOTIC
MONOCHORIONIC

fused

DIAMNIOTIC
DICHORIONIC

MONOAMNIOTIC
MONOCHORIONIC

forked cord

PLACENTATION
OF TWINS

double
monster

(one cord)

Fig. 6.3. Placentation of twins. From Strong and Corney (1967) by permission of the authors and Pergamon Press Ltd.

VASCULAR COMMUNICATIONS

Perhaps the greatest difference between monochorionic and dichorionic twins is that the former share a blood circulation whilst the latter rarely have any blood in common. This can have far reaching implications. In monochorionic twins the most powerful intrauterine influences determining growth are often related to the intertwin haemodynamics and this may also apply to malformations (see p.48). In dichorionic pairs, on the other hand, the sites of implantation of the two placentae are probably of paramount importance.

Monochorionic Placentae

For several centuries it had been known that communicating vessels occur in monochorionic placentae (Smellie 1752) and in 1870 Hyrtl demonstrated all the, now well recognized, types and combinations of anastomoses—the superficial arterio-arterial and veno-venous and the deep (parenchymatous) arteriovenous. Schatz (1900) went on to confirm this work and then focused his attention on the deep arterio-venous anastomoses. He gave much thought to the effects on the fetus of this shared or, as he called it, 'third circulation' (the first two being the fetal circulations of each twin). It was not until the 1960s that interest was revived (Corney 1966; Benirschke and Driscoll 1967; Strong and Corney 1967).

It is now generally accepted that most, if not all, monochorionic placentae have at least one type of anastomosis of which arterio-arterial, often combined with arterio-venous, is the commonest (Benirschke and Driscoll 1967; Strong and Corney 1967; Cameron 1968; Boyd and Hamilton 1970). Superficial anastomoses can often be seen with the naked eye but the patterns can be determined accurately only by injection studies.

Similar communicating channels exist in monochorionic monoamniotic placentae (Wharton et al. 1968; Bhargava 1976), although not invariably (Benirschke and Driscoll 1967; Strong and Corney 1967).

The Fetofetal Transfusion Syndrome
When no superficial anastomoses are present to compensate for the arteriovenous blood flow a chronic haemodynamic imbalance may

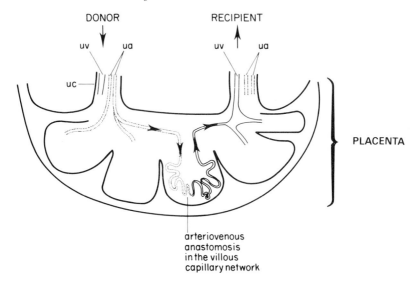

Fig. 6.4. The arteriovenous anastomosis present in the chronic form of fetofetal transfusion syndrome. uc = umbilical cord, uv = umbilical vein, ua = umbilical artery.

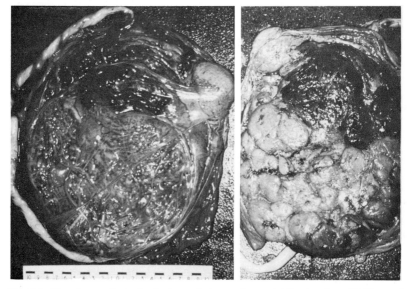

Fig. 6.5. The placenta in the fetofetal transfusion syndrome. (a) Fetal surface. (b) Maternal surface. The donor portion is large and pale while the recipient portion is engorged and smaller. By permission of Mr. J. Erskine.

develop between monochorionic twins (Fig. 6.4). This results in the fetofetal transfusion syndrome. One fetus transfuses the other via arterio-venous anastomoses and causes anaemia to himself (see Fig. 7.2), the donor, and polycythaemia to the recipient. The outcome is often disastrous for both.

The appearance of the placenta in this condition is striking and characteristic (Fig. 6.5). The recipient's portion is deeply coloured

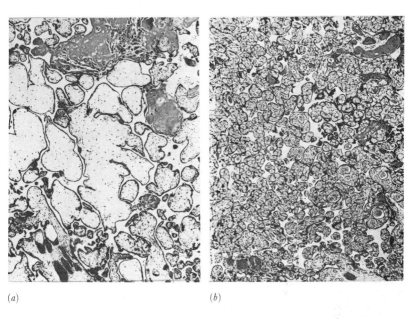

(*a*) (*b*)

Fig. 6.6. The histology of the placenta in the fetofetal transfusion syndrome. (a) Donor—the chorionic villi are bulky and fetal vessels are scarcely visible. (b) Recipient—fetal capillaries are numerous and engorged with blood. From Strong and Corney (1967) by permission of the authors and Pergamon Press.

and is often smaller with dilated engorged blood vessels. The histology, however, is unremarkable and normal for the period of gestation. In contrast, the donor's portion is pale and bulky with a high placental:fetal ratio. On microscopy the chorionic villi are oedematous and pleomorphic. The two layers of the trophoblast are thicker and well preserved and syncytial knots are scarce. The fetal capillaries are often filled with nucleated cells (Fig. 6.6). Some authors have compared the appearance with that found in the placentae of rhesus-sensitized infants (Benirschke and Driscoll

1967) but Aherne et al. (1968) in their detailed morphometric studies found that the characteristic villous hyperplasia did not occur. They showed that both the volume and surface area of the chorionic tissue were much greater in the donor twin. They thought, however, that this was due to oedematous swelling alone. The total volume and surface area of the fetal capillary beds in the two territories were similar but, as the capillary diameter in that of the donor was sometimes only half that of the recipient, these capillaries must be much longer.

Little is known about the function of this grossly abnormal placenta but Aherne et al. (1968) thought that the donor fetus might well receive less nourishment that his twin. This could be due, in part, to a reduction in maternofetal transfer across the abnormal placental basement membrane but he suggested that it may also be due to a sluggish blood flow in the narrow, elongated fetal capillaries of this part of the placenta. The low levels of the maternally derived protein IgG found in newborn donor twins provide further evidence of a disturbance in maternofetal transfer (Bryan 1976; Bryan et al. 1976).

The great majority of cases of the transfusion syndrome have diamniotic placentation, but several instances of the syndrome in monoamniotic twins have been reported (Rausen et al. 1965; Meyer et al. 1970; Pochedly and Musiker 1970).

Dichorionic Placentae

Although common in some animals vascular communications in dichorionic placentae in man are extremely rare (Benirschke and Driscoll 1967; Strong and Corney 1967; Corney 1975*b*). Many earlier reports are of dubious accuracy. Cameron (1968) however, reported two authentic cases from the Birmingham Twin Study in both of which the twins were probably MZ. The previously mentioned case of unlike sex twins with only a remnant of septal chorion had visible vascular communications and blood examination showed chimerism (Nylander and Osunkoya 1970) (see p.48).

There have been no satisfactorily proven examples of the fetofetal transfusion syndrome in dichorionic placentae. Those cases in which it has been suspected (Michaels 1967; Allen 1972) did not have injection studies. It may well be that the twin was anaemic for other reasons such as a fetomaternal haemorrhage (Strong and Corney 1967; Bryan 1976).

EXAMINATION OF THE PLACENTA

In 1961 Benirschke wrote a paper entitled 'Accurate recording of twin placentation. A plea to the Obstetrician'. His plea has been echoed since to both obstetricians and paediatricians (Strong and Corney 1967; Corney 1975*b*). By many it remains unheeded. The placenta may receive but a cursory glance; information which is vital to long-term twin studies, let alone of help in the immediate care of a sick baby, is all too often consigned to the incinerator. Comments in the medical records frequently give no indication of the placental membranes and remarks such as 'single' and 'binovular' are misleading.

As soon as the first twin is delivered the cord should be labelled according to the hospital practice. This will vary between hospitals but must remain consistent within; confusion arises if obstetricians adopt individual methods. Probably the most satisfactory and logical practice is to give the first cord a single clamp (or tape) and the second two clamps on the grounds that only standard (and readily available) equipment need be used.

After delivery of the placenta the site of insertion of the cords should be described and any anomalies or discrepancy in thickness and length noted. If an umbilical artery is missing the paediatrician should be informed.

Samples of cord blood for zygosity determination should be collected (taking care to avoid contamination with maternal blood) into heparinized bottles clearly labelled 'Twin 1' and 'Twin 2'. Clotted blood can also provide useful, although more limited, information. These samples should be stored at 4°C (not frozen) until sent together with similar samples from both parents, if possible, for testing of genetic markers (see p.25). If placental tissue is also required (see p.25) a full-thickness block of placenta (about 10 g) should be taken from diametrically opposed sites and stored at -20°C (unless immediate facilities for examination are available). If injection studies of the placental vessels (see below) are planned this specimen should be taken later.

If the placentae are separate or easily separable they should be weighed individually. Fused dichorionic and monochorionic placentae will obviously be weighed as one. If there is a clear demarcation between the two territories a rough estimation of the relative size of the two portions should be made. Note that the septum is not necessarily an indication of the territorial boundaries as injection studies have shown that often the two do not coincide

(Strong and Corney 1967; Fig. 6.7). Diagrams are helpful and should be used routinely.

The most important part of the examination of the twin placenta is the relationships of the membranes; these should be examined gently to avoid tearing. Characteristically the amnion is more transparent and friable than the chorion and can readily be stripped from the placenta leaving a smooth surface (of chorion).

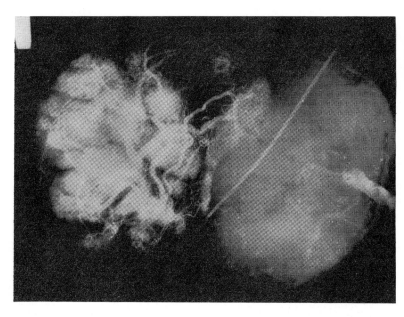

Fig. 6.7. X-ray of fused dichorionic placentae. One placenta has been injected with contrast medium. A catheter lies along the base of the septum showing that the junction of the vascular territories does not correspond to the insertion of the septum. From Strong and Corney (1967) by permission of the authors and Pergamon Press.

The amnions should peel right back to the umbilical cords and form a collar at their bases. No septum will then remain in monochorionic placentae whereas in dichorionic a single (fused) or two separate layers of chorion persist. The chorion is more opaque (Figs. 6.8 and 6.9) and cannot be separated from the placenta, except by tearing, as it is an integral part of the placental tissue. The chorionic ridge at the base of the septum is a good clue to a dichorionic placenta (Bleisch 1964). Occasionally difficulty arises if

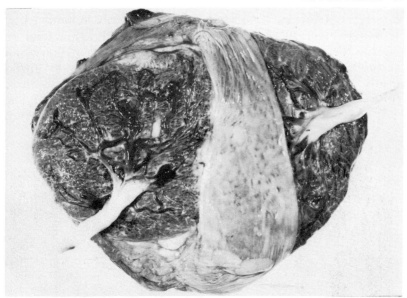

Fig. 6.8. Fused dichorionic diamniotic placenta. From Strong and Corney (1967) by permission of the authors and Pergamon Press.

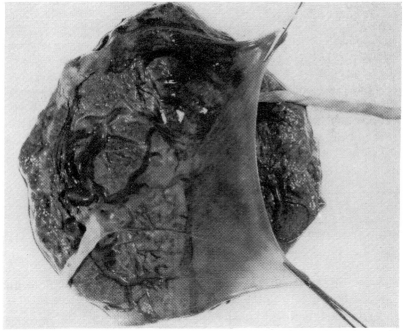

Fig. 6.9. Monochorionic diamniotic placenta. From Strong and Corney (1967) by permission of the authors and Pergamon Press.

the septal membranes are fused and this can only be resolved by histology (Fig. 6.10). For full details of histological examination see Bourne (1962). Usually, however, macroscopic examination by an experienced observer is as reliable as histology (Nylander 1970*c*;

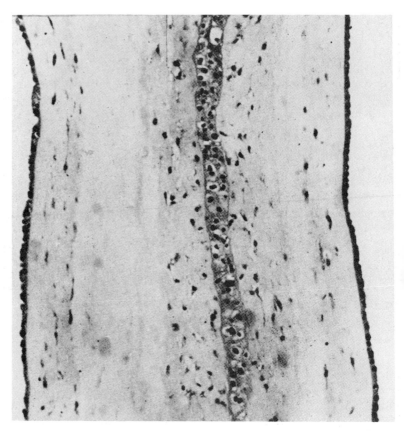

Fig. 6.10. The dividing membrane of a fused dichorionic placenta. The two outer layers are composed of amnion. Between them the two layers of chorion have fused in the mid-line. (H & E × 34). From Strong and Corney (1967) by permission of the authors and Pergamon Press.

Corney 1975*b*) and the latter needs only to be done in doubtful cases.

Accurate identification of vascular anastomoses will rarely be required for clinical purposes. Injection studies are usually confined to research projects. However, the techniques are (usually) not difficult to apply and the result can be both informative and decorative (Fig. 6.11). Those interested should gain experience on 'straightforward' specimens before a complicated case presents itself. Many coloured liquids (including red wine) have been

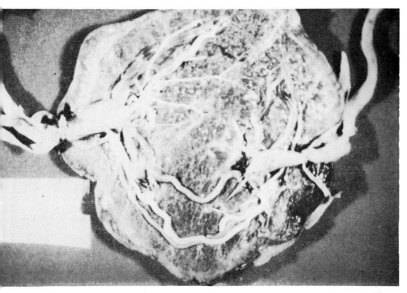

Fig. 6.11. Monochorionic diamniotic placenta. The vessels of twin 2 (right) have been injected and the vessels of the other twin have filled through both arterial and venous anastomoses. From Strong and Corney (1967) by permission of the authors and Pergamon Press.

injected to demonstrate placental vessels and their communications. Full details are given in Strong and Corney's (1967) beautifully illustrated book on *The Twin Placenta* as well as by others (Benirschke and Driscoll 1967). The use of radiopaque materials has enabled fascinating x-ray studies to be made (Strong and Corney 1967; Aherne et al. 1968; Fig. 6.12). For the practitioner who just wishes to demonstrate the existence and types of communicating channels, milk or coloured saline are the simplest and most readily available media. If the vessels are intact, all the blood can be washed out through catheters inserted into the vessels of the umbilical cords. If they are torn or examination has been delayed, then particular areas can be catheterized and examined separately.

Quantitative morphological studies of twin placentae are well described by Aherne and his colleagues (Aherne and Dunnill 1966;

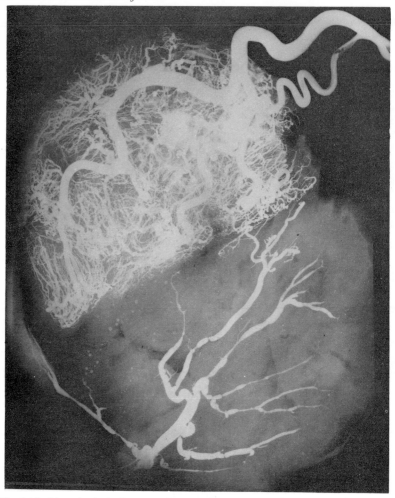

Fig. 6.12. Monochorionic diamniotic placenta. Contrast medium has been injected through the umbilical arteries of twin 2 and flowed through an arterial anastomosis of twin 1. It has just begun to fill its umbilical arteries in retrograde manner. From Strong and Corney (1967) by permission of the authors and Pergamon Press.

Aherne et al. 1968) but are research procedures and are beyond the scope of this book. More detailed descriptions of the examination of the placenta in general are given elsewhere (Benirschke and Driscoll 1967; Strong and Corney 1967; Boyd and Hamilton 1970; Corney 1975*b*; Fox 1978).

7. Newborn Twins

The birth of twins always causes excitement in the delivery room but is also bound to cause some anxiety. The complications that may arise during the labour and delivery of twins have already been discussed (see Chapter 5). Because of the risk of these complications and of prematurity two members of the paediatric staff should be present whenever possible. Two full sets of equipment for resuscitation must always be available.

LENGTH OF GESTATION

The average length of a twin pregnancy is about 260 days—3 weeks shorter than for singletons (MacGillivray 1975b). Between 20 and 30% of twins are born before the 37th week and are, therefore, preterm. The reasons for the shorter gestation are still uncertain (see p.62). In many cases, however, it would be a disadvantage to the twin fetus to continue intrauterine life to term. Uteroplacental function seems to be suboptimal during the last few weeks in many twin pregnancies. This is suggested by the rapidly increasing discrepancy in weights between twins and singletons as they approach term (Fig. 7.1) and by the rising perinatal mortality rate after 38–39 weeks gestation (Stucki et al. 1982).

Poor placental function may also explain why MZ twins tend to have a shorter gestation than DZ (Weekes et al. 1977a; MacGillivray 1982). The 'third circulation' may well reduce the efficiency of maternofetal transfer still further.

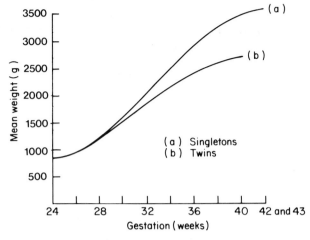

Fig. 7.1. Birth weights of twins and singletons in relation to gestational age. From McGillivray (1975c) by permission of the author and W.B. Saunders Co. Ltd.

Assessment of Gestational Age

The gestational age of the newborn baby can be assessed by certain neurological and physical criteria. This is now well-established practice with singletons (Dubowitz et al. 1970). Recent studies have shown the same criteria to be equally appropriate in twins (Keet et al. 1974; Woods and Malan 1977). Twins with only small intrapair differences in weight tend to have more similar scores to their co-twin than those with large weight discrepancies. Although the lighter twin has similar scores on neurological criteria he tends to have a lower score than his twin on physical criteria (Woods and Malan 1977). The pattern shown by the lighter twin is similar to that of an intrauterine growth-retarded singleton.

In his study of 33 pairs of twins Keet et al. (1974) found that there was no significant difference in the mean combined neurological and physical score between the heavier and lighter babies. However, in the group with large weight discrepancies (over 15%) only three out of 12 lighter twins had a higher score than their co-twin.

BIRTH WEIGHT

About half of newborn twins weigh less than 2.5 kg (Potter 1963) which is over seven times the incidence in singletons (Merkatz

1979). As well as being of low birth weight many of these infants, particularly the more mature, are light for their gestational age when compared with singletons (Fig. 7.1). Indeed the optimal birth weight for twins appears to be between 2.5 and 3.5 kg whereas for singletons it is between 3.5 and 4 kg (Butler and Alberman 1969). As in singletons, male twin infants tend to be heavier than females (Parsons 1965; Corey et al. 1979).

In twins with large intrapair discrepancies in weight the heavier infant is usually appropriately grown for its gestational age when compared with singletons. The lighter infant, on the other hand, must have suffered from intrauterine growth retardation and is at all the risks of a small-for-dates baby, in particular that of hypoglycaemia (Reisner et al. 1965).

The birth weight of twins appears to be unrelated to birth order. Most recent studies have found no significant differences in weight between the first- and secondborn. Earlier studies tended to show that the firstborn was heavier but the difference is removed when macerated stillbirths, which are nearly always both smaller and secondborn, are excluded from the sample.

The problems of low birth weight and of prematurity are many and the reader is referred to textbooks on neonatal medicine for guidance on their management. Mention here will be made of disorders which are either peculiar to or have particular expression (e.g. intrapair differences) in twins.

RESPIRATORY DISTRESS SYNDROME

Respiratory distress due to hyaline membrane disease is common in twins due to their high incidence of prematurity. Neither zygosity nor sex of the twins have been shown to influence the incidence of respiratory distress syndrome (Myrianthopoulos 1970). However, it would not be surprising to find the disease more commonly occurring in MZ twins in view of their higher rate of prematurity. Concordance appears to be higher in MZ than DZ twins and it has been suggested that there may be a genetic determinant to the disorder (Myrianthopoulos et al. 1971). On the other hand if the babies are of shorter gestation it is more likely that both would be affected. When one twin alone is affected it is almost always the secondborn. Likewise, if both are affected the second is more severely so (Potter 1963). Butler and Alberman (1969) found that significantly more secondborn infants died from hyaline membrane disease and the risk was increased further in those with a birth interval of over 30 minutes. Perinatal anoxia is almost certainly a contributory factor to the secondborn's increased susceptibility to respiratory distress syndrome.

On the other hand other influences may give the leading twin a positive advantage. It is well known that some stresses such as prolonged rupture of the membranes reduce the risk of respiratory distress syndrome and two such cases have been reported in twins (Rajegowda et al. 1975). Chorioamnionitis, without rupture of membranes, is commoner in the sac of the first twin (see p.56). This may cause stress which would promote the production of phospholipids and thereby protect the infant from hyaline membrane disease.

The phospholipid profile of a fetus may determine the management of a preterm labour or the timing of an elective caesarean section. Yet there is still uncertainty as to whether levels differ between the first and second twin. Obladen and Gluck (1977) found that surfactant phospholipids were invariably lower in the affected twin and in the vaginally delivered twins this was always the secondborn. Likewise Weller et al. (1976) found that the firstborn of two sets of triplets had much higher phospholipid levels than the succeeding babies. Jenkins and Baum (1981) in their study of lecithin:sphyngomyelin (L:S) ratios in pharyngeal aspirates, found no general trend to suggest that the lungs of the first twin were more mature than those of the secondborn. However, there was no case in which the first had an immature L:S ratio or developed hyaline membrane disease when the second was mature.

Several workers have found no intrapair differences in phospholipids in amniotic fluid taken before the onset of labour (Sims et al. 1976; Spellacy et al. 1977; Norman and Joubert 1982) whereas the leading twin had a significantly higher L:S ratio in cases of emergency caesarean section after a period of labour. These findings suggest that as long as the sample is taken before the onset of labour amniotic fluid from one sac is sufficient to predict the lung maturity of both fetuses.

HAEMOGLOBIN LEVELS

Neither zygosity nor birth order appear to affect the level of haemoglobin in the cord bloods of twins (Bryan 1976). Intrapair discrepancies, once the cases of fetofetal transfusion syndrome have been excluded, are also similar in DZ and MZ twins (Kauppila et al. 1975; Bryan 1976). Abraham (1969), however, suggests that the first of MZ twins may be depleted of blood due to interfetal shunting during delivery. Although he found no difference in haemoglobin levels at birth, by 24 hours of age the firstborn had significantly lower levels.

In dichorionic twins Clemetson (1956) found that cord haemoglobin levels were significantly higher in the lighter twin and suggested that this may be due to relative intrauterine hypoxia. Polycythaemia is well recognized in association with intrauterine growth retardation in singletons.

In addition to the known causes of anaemia in the newborn, monochorionic twins may be anaemic as a result of their shared intrauterine circulation. The donor twin of both the acute (see p.65) and chronic fetofetal transfusion syndrome (see p.46 and

Table 7.1. Characteristic features of the two forms of fetofetal transfusion syndrome

		Acute	*Chronic*
Cause	Placenta	Arterio-arterial or veno-venous transfusion	Arterio-venous transfusion
Pregnancy	Ultrasound	Normal	Diverging BPD
	Amniotic fluid	Normal volume	Polyhydramnios
Placenta	Appearance	Normal	d—Pale, bulky, oedematous r—Engorged
	Vascular anastomoses	Visible superficial	Invisible arterio-venous
	Histology	Normal	d—Trophoblast immaturity r—Normal
Infants	Birth weight	Similar	r—Heavier than d
	Blood film	Normal	d—Erythroblastosis r—Normal
	Complications	d—Shock++ CCF++ Anaemia+ r—CCF++ Polycythaemia+ Jaundice+	d—Birth asphyxia+ Anaemia++ CCF± Small-for-dates r—Polycythaemia++ Jaundice+ CCF±

Key: d = donor
    r = recipient
    BPD = biparietal diameter
    CCF = congestive cardiac failure

Table 7.1) and a single survivor with disseminated intravascular coagulation (see p.59) are two examples of this.

The Chronic Fetofetal Transfusion Syndrome

An intrapair discrepancy in cord blood haemoglobin levels of over 5 g/100 ml has been suggested as the diagnostic criterion for the fetofetal transfusion syndrome. Rausen et al. (1965) found no discrepancy of such magnitude in a series of DZ twins, all of whom would be expected to have dichorionic placentation. As haemoglobin concentrations may not be available for infants who die before, or soon after, delivery, a combination of other criteria, such as polyhydramnios in one sac, large birthweight discrepancies, and characteristic placental histology will often be needed in making the diagnosis.

Even when haemoglobin levels are available they should not be used as the only criteria for the diagnosis as they will not distinguish the fetofetal transfusion syndrome from other causes of anaemia in one twin. Intrapartum blood loss or fetomaternal haemorrhage, for instance, could both result in large intrapair discrepancies in haemoglobin level.

Extreme examples of intrapair haematological differences have been described: haemoglobin discrepancies exceeding 20 g% (Bosma 1954; Klingberg et al. 1955; Sacks 1959), individual haemoglobin levels greater than 30 g% (Bosma 1954; Sacks 1959), and alarmingly high haematocrit levels. In Sack's (1959) case the haematocrit of one twin who survived apparently unscathed was 93%. At the other extreme donor twins have survived haemoglobin levels of less than 4 g% (Klingberg et al. 1955; Shorland 1971). Even with smaller discrepancies in haemoglobin levels there may be striking differences in the blood films of the two infants—a normoblastaemia being evident in that of the donor (Strong and Corney 1967).

Nutrients are of course transfused together with the haemoglobin and it is not surprising that the recipient twin is usually much heavier than the donor (Fig. 7.2). Studies of protein chemistry have shown much higher levels of all proteins in the recipient (Kloosterman 1963; Bryan 1976; Bryan et al. 1976). The donor twin may have very low levels of total proteins and albumin and, presumably, colloid osmotic pressure (Bryan 1976). Hydrops fetalis has occasionally been reported in both recipient and donor but it is surprising that this is not more common particularly in the donor

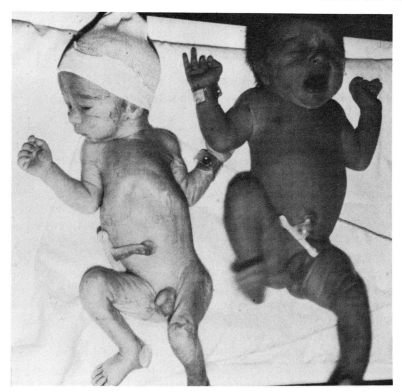

Fig. 7.2. The fetofetal transfusion syndrome showing intrauterine growth retardation and pallor of the donor (weight 1.6 kg Hb 7.9 g/100 ml) and plethora of recipient (weight 2.7 kg, Hb 21 g/100 ml).

in view of the profound anaemia and hypoalbuminaemia. However, some infants who are free from oedema at birth may become severely oedematous within a few days (Bryan and Slavin 1974).

Management
The chronic fetofetal transfusion syndrome is rarely diagnosed before delivery although the presence of polyhydramnios in a multiple pregnancy should always raise the suspicion. In mild cases the diagnosis is often missed or made only because of the result of a routine blood count. Sometimes it is only because of a careful placental examination that the condition is suspected. Many of these infants need no special treatment. Others may be severely distressed. The donor twin, already embarrassed by chronic hypoxia from the anaemia, often suffers from severe birth asphyxia particularly if he is the secondborn.

As the fetuses have usually had time to compensate for their haemodynamic disturbances a blood transfusion is rarely urgent. Indeed a rapid transfusion to the donor may precipitate cardiac failure whereas a sudden withdrawal of blood from the recipient might, by reducing the blood volume, increase the dangers from the hyperviscosity of polycythaemia. Both infants may be in incipient or overt cardiac failure and this should be treated before transfusions are attempted. In order to avoid a sudden change in blood volume exchange transfusions are then the best treatment for both babies. Theoretically an intertwin transfusion should be the method of choice and this has been done successfully (Valaes and Doxiadis 1960). In practice, however, the difficulties of coping with two, often very sick, babies together, either of whom might suddenly need resuscitation, usually precludes this apparently logical practice.

Thus the donor should be given a slow exchange transfusion with fresh partially packed blood. It is unnecessary and potentially dangerous fully to correct the anaemia immediately. One or more top-up transfusions can always be given later. His iron stores are likely to be severely depleted due to loss of fetal haemoglobin. Iron supplements may be necessary for several months.

Blood viscosity rises rapidly when the haematocrit in venous blood reaches 70% (or 75% in capillary blood). An exchange plasma or albumin transfusion should be considered in all recipient twins with levels higher than this.

The donor twin should be treated as a small-for-dates baby and a careful watch kept for complications such as hypoglycaemia and hypothermia. As he often has a deficiency of the maternally derived immunoglobulin G (Bryan 1976; Bryan et al. 1976) the donor twin could be particularly vulnerable to infections. Although there have been several case reports of donor twins having severe infections in the first 6 months (Herlitz 1941; Perez and Gallo 1965; Abraham 1967; Bryan and Slavin 1974) no controlled study has been reported. The recipient, although well nourished, has no less hazardous a start in life. The consequences of untreated polycythaemia can be disastrous. Sludging of the blood may produce vascular thrombi which will, according to their sites, have serious effects such as convulsions or neurological damage from cerebral vascular occlusions or renal failure due to renal vessel occlusion.

Hyperbilirubinaemia, often difficult to detect in a plethoric infant, can develop with alarming speed as the large load of haemoglobin is broken down. Frequent checks on serum bilirubin are mandatory.

The Acute Fetofetal Transfusion Syndrome (see p.65)

An exsanguinated donor twin may be one of the most urgent emergencies encountered in the delivery room. In a shocked baby the significance of the pallor is easily missed but other resuscitative measures will be of no avail until the hypovolaemia, sometimes severe, is corrected with a transfusion of blood or other plasma expander. Likewise the recipient may need urgent reduction of his increased blood volume, if cardiac failure is to be averted, by withdrawal of blood from the umbilical vein.

Cord haemoglobin levels are often misleading in the acute form of fetofetal transfusion syndrome. They may be normal with no intrapair discrepancy. Measurements taken 6–12 hours later when the intravascular circulation has reached equilibrium with the other fluid compartments of the body, often show much greater intrapair discrepancies than the initial samples.

Distinction between the acute and chronic forms of fetofetal transfusion syndrome is rarely difficult (Klebe and Ingomar 1972; Tan et al. 1979; Table 7.1). In the chronic form infants invariably have discrepancies in body weight, characteristic macroscopic and microscopic changes in the placenta (see p.77) and an erythroblastotic blood film in the donor.

Disseminated Intravascular Coagulation

If one monochorionic twin dies in utero thromboplastin may enter the circulation of the surviving fetus and cause disseminated intravascular coagulation, resulting in tissue necrosis and haemorrhage. In those that survive long enough, severe anaemia may develop (see p.59). It is perhaps surprising that this disorder is not more common in single surviving twins.

PERINATAL MORTALITY

Despite improvements in both obstetric and neonatal care the risks to the twin fetus and newborn remain at least three times that for a singleton. In the 1970s the perinatal mortality rates of twins in Western countries lay between 80 and 125 per 1000 (Farooqui et al. 1973; Laursen 1973; Dawood et al. 1975; Kauppila et al. 1975; Khoo and Green 1975; Weekes et al. 1977b; Hoffman et al. 1978; Ellis et al. 1979; Merkatz 1979). Lower figures are now emerging

(Stucki et al. 1982). The main contributor to the high toll is prematurity and its complications. It is therefore not surprising to find that the increase in neonatal deaths in twins is proportionately greater than fetal deaths. Potter (1963) found that intrauterine death was twice as common in twins as in singletons whereas deaths in the neonatal period were increased fivefold. Other problems specific to a multiple pregnancy increase the perinatal mortality rate further. These other factors include fetal malpresentation and dystocia, the complications of a shared fetal circulation in monochorionic twins and the higher incidence of lethal malformations.

Many studies have shown a higher perinatal mortality rate amongst MZ than DZ twins (Potter 1963; Ferguson 1964; Behrman 1965; Benirschke and Driscoll 1967; Myrianthopoulos 1970) and amongst like-sexed than unlike-sexed twins (Guttmacher and Kohl 1958).

Benirschke and Kim (1973) found a 26% mortality rate in monochorionic twins compared with a 9% in dichorionic. The higher rate amongst this group of MZ twins is not surprising and the dangers of the third circulation have already been discussed. It might be expected that MZ twins with dichorionic placentation would have the same mortality rate as DZ twins as they are subject to the same environmental influences. However, Corney et al. (1972) have shown that MZ dichorionic twins grow less well than their DZ counterparts so it may well be that all MZ twins are at a disadvantage compared with DZ.

Boys fare worse than girls regardless of zygosity. Fujikura and Froelich (1971) found that the highest perinatal mortality rate was amongst male–male pairs. In unlike-sexed pairs Butler and Alberman (1968) found that if the male was firstborn in a pair of unlike sex then his risk of death was similar to his secondborn sister, whereas if the infants were born in the reverse order the boy had twice the mortality rate of the girl.

MOTHER–INFANT BONDING

Even if both twins are well and able to be with their mother from the start, the mother of twins will need particular support and understanding. This need will be even greater if one or both babies are ill and separated from her. For most mothers bonding to one baby is a full-time preoccupation both emotionally and physically. Bonding to two can be an enormous strain.

It is well recognized that mothers find it more difficult to relate to babies from whom they have been separated during the first days following delivery than to those who have been with them from the start. Klaus and Kennell (1970) have shown the importance of early physical contact between a mother and her baby. With twins the firstborn, usually stronger, baby is often handed straight to the mother. She may, however, get only a glimpse of the second baby before it is whisked away to an incubator. If this happens it is easy for the mother to 'forget' that she has another baby. She should be encouraged to handle the other baby and see as much of him as his condition can possibly allow. If necessary arrangements should be made for the mother to visit this baby in the special care baby unit as soon as she is ready to leave the delivery room. In many cases it may be wise to send both babies to the unit together (preferably with the mother as well) in order to reduce the problems of separation.

Eye-to-eye contact is also vital to mother–infant bonding. Robson and Moss (1970) have demonstrated how it initiates or releases care-taking responses in the mother. If one twin is visually more responsive than the other it may, without the mother realizing, receive more of her attention. Even if she responds to both equally she is bound to find it harder to give her concentration to each when there will often be simultaneous demands for her attention.

Many more mothers of twins than singletons have to cope with the acute emotional crisis caused by the birth of a premature baby. This seems to be unavoidable even when every effort is made to reduce the separation of the baby from the mother (Blake et al. 1975). The very fact of producing a premature baby, even a healthy one, is for most mothers an extremely distressing experience. They may find it particularly difficult to handle their (mixed) feelings if one baby is thriving and the other is critically ill.

Many mothers easily tell their twins apart. Others find it much more difficult. Some may be distressed by the confusion and this may impede their ability to bond to each individual baby. The mother (and the nursing staff) should be encouraged to identify the babies at all times and to call them by their names. Each cot should be recognizable at a distance and the babies themselves easily distinguishable by, for instance, the different colours of clothes.

NAMING TWINS

Clearly the choosing of names for a baby is a matter deeply personal to the parents. Approval or otherwise is not the responsibility of the medical or nursing staff. Nevertheless the implications for a child or adult of being landed with a 'twin' name can be tactfully pointed out. Even now, when parents, on the whole, are more aware of the importance of allowing twins to develop as individuals, the temptation to give rhyming names, such as Sita and Gita, or like-sounding such as Jean and Jane or Dean and Darren, seems hard to resist. Similar names for opposite sexes such as Robert and Roberta, or Dellis and Dennis, cause added confusion. Even the same initial can be a disadvantage to teenagers not least with personal correspondence.

ADOPTION

In the past twins were often separated for adoption. Fortunately most, if not all, adoption agencies now place twins together. This is at least the practice with healthy babies and few would dispute that this is right.

Despite the difficulties of mothering twins and the disadvantages to the twins themselves it seems wrong to separate children who have developed so closely before birth. A single surviving twin often appears to miss his partner even if that baby dies at birth. Furthermore, a sadness for many adopted children is that of having no true (blood) relations. A twin or other sibling can greatly enhance their sense of security.

There is more disagreement about what should be done if one baby is ill or handicapped. A number of questions are bound to arise. Should the chances of a successful placement for the healthy baby be jeopardized or delayed? Should a child be burdened with a handicapped sibling when this can be avoided? Although there is no shortage of adoptive parents for a single baby or even for a healthy pair of twins, handicapped babies are much harder to place. Despite these obvious problems, however, many people— particularly parents of twins—feel that the babies should remain together. Apart from other considerations the healthy twin may sooner or later feel a heavy guilt for having 'deserted' his needy sibling. There need be no delay in placing the normal baby with the intended adopting parents and the other twin can then follow as soon as he is fit enough.

Parents who are considering adopting twins need special counselling. They must have realistic guidance as to the emotional and physical demands of two babies. In addition it is obviously important that they clarify their own motives for adopting two babies and make sure that the mere attraction of twins is not a significant consideration.

Adoption agencies provide information and many arrange group meetings for prospective parents. The Twins Clubs Association has a register of families with adopted twins and many of the parents are happy to talk to prospective parents as well as social workers and other professionals involved with the adoption.

GOING HOME

In hospital the mother of twins is the centre of attention and the successful candidate for any extra help and support that is available. She is told how lucky she is to have two babies and usually feels this to be true. Rarely is she given any constructive preparation for the tasks that lie ahead.

In the United Kingdom a family with twins does not automatically qualify for extra practical assistance (e.g. a home help). Thus everything possible should be done to help the family prepare realistically for the months to come; to organize in advance the help that is available; to invest from the start in any time-saving devices that can be afforded, to ensure that the family doctor and health visitor are alerted to the family's need for support (Linney 1983).

Many mothers are ill advised on equipment for twins and have no access to a source of secondhand articles. Many waste money by automatically buying everything in duplicate. Maternity units should keep close contact with twins' families in the area, usually through the local twins club. Should the new mother wish it, a member is always happy to visit and advise on types and sources of equipment. The mother of undiagnosed twins particularly benefits from this service.

Some twins clubs actually store their equipment and first-size clothes in the hospital. Parents then have a wide range readily available. For pregnant mothers it is wise to encourage them to book, rather than buy, the pram. The business of selling a twin pram, if one baby dies, can be particularly distressing.

As the father has of necessity a more important role to play in the care of twins, the earlier he can be encouraged to do this the better. Even the most supportive may be apprehensive about handling a very small baby. His confidence will be greatly increased with practice under supervision in the hospital.

Often one baby is ready to go home before the other. If the discharge of the second has to be delayed for several weeks then separation from both mother and the other baby will be hard to avoid. Where at all possible, however, it is best for both to be kept together. The notion that it is easier to start with one baby alone seems to be ill-founded. It is all the harder to adapt to two babies if a routine with one has already been established. Furthermore if the mother is busy at home with one baby she often finds it difficult to visit the other. She becomes increasingly attached to the one she is with and may find it hard to accept the second baby.

One single mother of a 3-kg girl and a 1.5-kg boy went home after 10 days with her daughter. She rarely visited the little boy, who had many neonatal problems. When he finally went home after 2 months she admitted to great difficulty in feeling any affection for him. It was over a year before she even began to accept him as she did her daughter. Another baby whose discharge had been delayed much longer than her twin brother was admitted later suffering from non-accidental injury.

When separation of the babies is unavoidable the mother should be strongly encouraged to visit the one remaining in hospital. Transport may be needed and a nursery and feeds for the twin must be available so that he can always be brought too, thus allowing the mother to spend long periods in the hospital without worrying about the other baby.

Older siblings will also need special consideration. They may well have been separated from their mother for several weeks if she was in hospital before delivery. After the birth the twins are often the overwhelming focus of attention. Siblings may well therefore feel rejected and insecure. These children should be with their mothers and the babies whenever possible.

8. Feeding Twins

For many mothers of older twins the blurred memory of the first 6 months of the babies' lives is of one endless round of feeding. Because of the enormous importance of establishing the easiest and most satisfactory feeding routine for both the mother and her twins a whole chapter is devoted to this subject.

BREAST-FEEDING

Many pairs of twins have been fully breast-fed and have thrived. Some have known no milk other than their mother's until after their first birthday (Addy 1975; Brewster 1979; Linney 1980a; Noble 1980; Stables 1980). It is well known that supply can equal demand: a healthy mother has a remarkable capacity to produce the required volume of milk, even enough to satisfy three babies (Noble 1980).

Despite this, many mothers of twins are still discouraged, even dissuaded, from breast-feeding on the fallacious grounds that they will be unlikely to have enough milk or that they will find it too tiring (Leonard 1959). In Addy's study of 173 mothers of twins, 12 were positively advised against breast-feeding and a further 15 assumed that it was not possible and were not enlightened until it was too late (Addy 1975).

There have, unfortunately, been few studies on feeding patterns in twins. In particular none have monitored the growth of those who were fed with breast milk. It is of practical importance to know how their growth compares with that of bottle-fed twins and of both breast- and bottle-fed singletons. The largest study is that of Addy (1975) in which 173 Californian mothers replied to written questionnaires. Forty-one of these mothers breast-fed their twins for varying lengths of time up to 10 months. The growth of these babies was said to be satisfactory but no measurements were taken.

Advantages

The advantages of breast-feeding are now well documented (Gunther 1973; Jelliffe and Jelliffe 1978). These include nutritional, immunological, psychological, practical and economic advantages. For a twin baby the benefits are even greater.

As many twins are born prematurely they are likely to be particularly vulnerable to infections. The immunological properties of breast milk give some protection against both bacterial and viral invasion. Mothers have more difficulty in bonding to premature infants, partly because of the inevitable separation if the baby has to be nursed on the special care baby unit. Studies have shown that

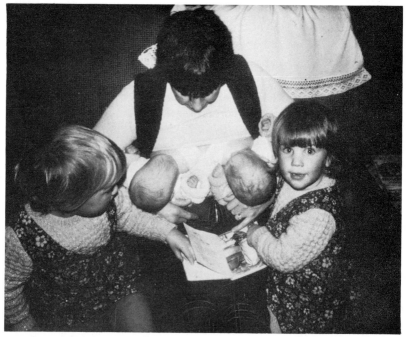

Fig. 8.1. Mother breast-feeding 6-month-old twin girls and entertaining the 2- and 3-year-old sisters at the same time.

mothers have fewer bonding problems if they breast-feed their babies so this may go some way to compensate for the separation.

Furthermore breast-feeding is the only way that a mother can feed and nurse both babies at the same time. As time is at a premium, and opportunities for cuddling much reduced, any means of providing the mother of twins with more nursing time should be welcomed (Fig. 8.1).

Finally the cost of powdered milks for two babies is considerable, particularly to a family budget which is already likely to be under strain. The recommended daily supplementation to the lactating mother's diet is 500 Kcal including 20 g of protein for each baby (National Academy of Sciences 1974). These extra requirements imposed by breast-feeding can be provided by relatively cheap foods. It has been calculated that the cost of supplementary foods need be no more than one-third of that of powdered milks (Jelliffe and Jelliffe 1975). In developing countries the additional hazards of overdilution and bacterial contamination of bottle feeds have been well documented (Muller 1976).

Disadvantages

The most obvious disadvantage of breast-feeding to the mother is that she can have no respite during the early months, when she will often be very tired. Breast-feeding two babies is also much more difficult to do discretely in public. Some mothers find this additional curtailment to a social life that is already much reduced a major disadvantage. Hopefully this particular disadvantage will soon be removed as social acceptance of the breast-feeding mother becomes more general.

Preparation

As soon as a multiple pregnancy is diagnosed the question of feeding should be discussed with the mother and the advantages of breast-feeding pointed out. Although a mother may have seen singletons being breast-fed, it is most unusual for her to have seen breast-feeding of twins; indeed some assume it is not possible and do not even consider the idea. Arrangements should therefore be made for the mother to visit another mother of twins at feed time (Fig. 8.2). Such a visit will always result in many queries being answered which might never even have been voiced in the antenatal clinic. Sometimes a lasting and supportive friendship will develop between the two mothers.

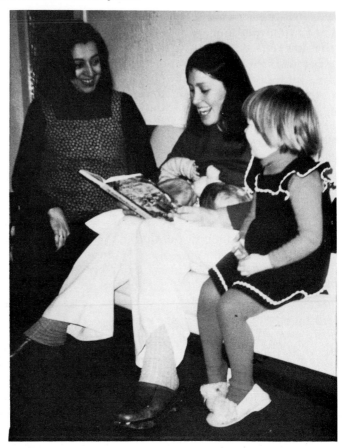

Fig. 8.2. Expectant mother of twins receiving advice on breast-feeding from mother of 5-month-old boys.

If the mother has already been admitted to hospital when twins are discovered then a visit to a mother in the postnatal ward is worthwhile. This is helpful for demonstrating the technique. However the memory of someone still feeding when the twins are several months old is more likely to give effective encouragement during the first, often difficult, weeks. Even a film or videotape (or at least photographs) of a mother breast-feeding twins can be both instructive and encouraging to an expectant mother if for some reason a personal visit is not possible.

The rate of successful breast-feeding of twins can be substantially increased with such antenatal education followed by support and encouragement when the babies arrive. In one maternity unit it was found that of 12 mothers who had planned to breast-feed their twins only one was successfully doing so after 6 weeks. Following the introduction of these more positive and supportive measures the number of mothers continuing to breast-feed after 6 weeks rose the following year to 11 out of 12 (Bryan 1977*b*).

Several studies have shown the importance in singletons of early suckling both for the establishment and for the continuation of breast-feeding (Salariya et al. 1978; Kennell et al. 1976). Although this is just as important, if not more so, in twins it is rare for both babies, or even one, to be put to the breast in the delivery room. The mother is more likely to have had a tiring and difficult delivery, the babies may be premature or suffer from birth asphyxia. All these factors make it more difficult to arrange for the twin infant to suckle early. Nevertheless far more twins could be safely put to the breast in the delivery room than is now the practice.

Techniques

The first decision is whether to feed the babies together or separately. There are advantages to both and a mother soon discovers which suits her best.

There appears to have been little work on the relative physiological advantages of the two methods. Tyson (1976) reports a higher prolactin response in mothers who suckle their twins simultaneously. It appears that the amount of prolactin released is a function both of the intensity of sucking and of the number of nipples stimulated. This suggests that, at least in the early days, when a full milk supply is still to be achieved, there are advantages in feeding both babies together.

If the babies are fed separately the mother can give her full concentration to each and she may find she is generally more comfortable. However, feeding times will take up a large portion of the day and she may also be distressed by the cries of the second hungry baby. Theoretically it is better to alternate the order for feeds. In practice the same baby often demands the food first. Either way a baby should be offered one breast only at a feed. Otherwise the first baby, by taking the fore-milk from both breasts, will receive milk with a much lower fat content than that of his twin.

The main advantage of feeding the babies together is the time saved, and time is a precious commodity. Some mothers find that it is actually more comfortable if both their breasts are emptying at

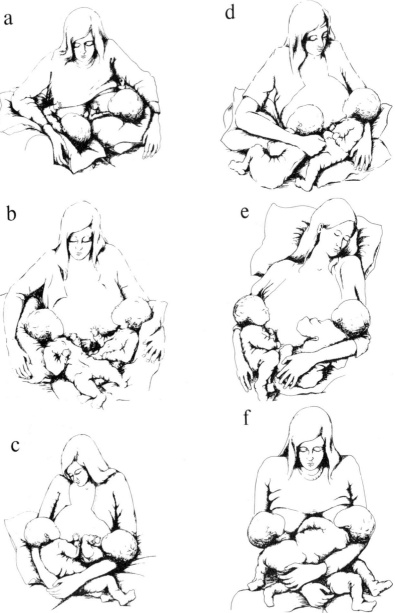

Fig. 8.3. Six positions for breast-feeding twins. (a) 'Football hold'. (b) Babies parallel to mother's body. (c) Babies criss-crossed and supported by pillows and mother's arms. (d) Babies facing same direction. (e) Mother in almost lying position and babies parallel to her body. (f) Babies are criss-crossed but supported only by mother's arms—suitable for 'emergency' feeds only. Drawn by Joan Moore.

the same time rather than having the feeling of tension in the overflowing unsucked breast.

The positioning of the babies during a feed is obviously a matter of personal preference. An astonishing number of different positions have been devised and some of these are illustrated here (Fig. 8.3). Most mothers tend to stick to one position but some may ring the changes.

The place for feeding is equally variable. Some mothers prefer to feed from their bed whenever feasible. The sofa with supportive cushions for the mother's back and pillows for the babies is popular, so is a large armchair. A recently produced triangular cushion, originally designed for patients sitting in bed, is an excellent support when reversed (i.e. in front of the mother), for both babies (Fig. 8.4).

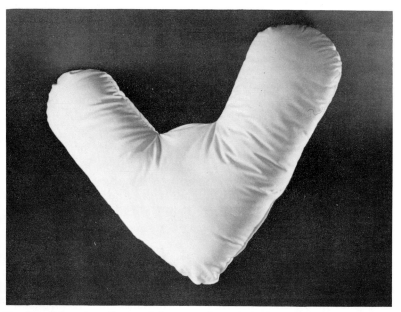

Fig. 8.4. Triangular pillow used for supporting twin babies during breast-feeding. By permission of J.D. Williams and Co. Ltd., The Dale St. Warehouses, Manchester X.

Most mothers prefer to change the babies' sides at each feed and have various ingenious methods of remembering who's due for which breast. A safety pin attached to a bra strap is a particular favourite, others keep daily charts. Still others trust to intuition and don't worry too much.

Some mothers find that the babies are happier on the same side each time and it has been claimed that they then regulate their own milk supply. Lopsidedness of the breasts is said to be a disadvantage of this method but I have yet to hear of this actually happening. In theory one-sided visual stimulation for such a large portion of a baby's waking hours could be detrimental to his development but as yet there is nothing to substantiate this idea.

As the advantages of demand feeding, rather than scheduled feeding to the clock, become more appreciated an increasing number of mothers of twins are choosing to feed their babies on demand. In Addy's (1975) study 78% of the babies were so fed. Any disturbance to the mother's routine seems to be offset by the advantages of having more contented babies.

A number of mothers find the most practical method is to feed both babies when one has indicated that he is hungry. This is particularly important at night so that the mother can avoid being woken again shortly afterwards.

Establishment of Breast-Feeding

Many mothers with just one baby have some difficulties with breast-feeding during the first few days. For mothers of twins the problems are proportionately greater and many find the first week a frustrating struggle.

The mother can be helped in many ways. In particular she should have the opportunity to suckle the babies in the delivery room and as often as she wishes to thereafter. Rest and minimum tension are essential. Both are difficult to provide for a mother with two babies to care for. The more help she can have with looking after the babies, the better. The father should be encouraged to help from the start.

Many mothers become frustrated and tearful if left to feed the two babies simultaneously on their own. In the early days it is often difficult to keep both babies attached to the breast. If one falls off the second may also be lost as the mother struggles to retrieve the first. If she resorts to feeding them separately her milk supply may be reduced, she becomes frustrated because the feeding round seems endless and a lactation crisis (Fig. 8.5) may set in.

It is most important that all mothers with twins should have someone by their side throughout the feed until they are entirely confident and choose to be left on their own. This need not be a highly qualified midwife. The father or an understanding friend can perform the task perfectly well.

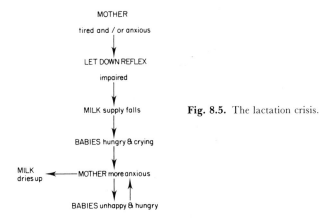

Fig. 8.5. The lactation crisis.

In some pairs of twins, particularly if there are large differences in weight between the two babies, one twin has a much stronger suck than the other. This can be a positive advantage to the weaker baby as his twin's stronger suck will invoke a let-down reflex in both breasts thereby supplying extra milk for both.

Problems

Lack of Encouragement

Many mothers complain not only of lack of information about breast-feeding twins but also of the negative approach of doctors and midwives. In many centres this attitude is changing but there is still need for more teaching on the particular problems of breast-feeding twins so that midwives can give more informed advice.

Many mothers find the postnatal ward, with its inflexible timetable, a harassing environment and because breast-feeding takes longer than bottle feeding they may resort to the latter in order to conform more easily to the rules of the ward.

Lack of Milk

Although supply should equal demand only too often the equilibrium is disturbed by the extraneous factors already mentioned. The babies may be premature and have an inadequate suck, the mother's anxiety may have reduced her prolactin response and the lactation crisis occurs (Fig. 8.5).

It is often difficult to decide if and when complementary feeds with cow's milk should be given. As many twins are small for dates and therefore at risk of hypoglycaemia these may be necessary sooner than would otherwise have been wished. Some mothers continue to give combined breast and bottle feeds for many months. Others alternate each feed, offering one baby the breast and the other the bottle. Occasionally a mother chooses to breast feed one entirely, usually the frailer, and bottle feed the other. This seems the least satisfactory practice as inevitably the mother will develop a much closer relationship with one baby than the other.

An innovation which may prove a great help to some mothers of twins is the Lact-Aid Nursing Supplementer (Avery 1972). This provides additional milk to the baby without interfering with sucking. The milk is supplied through a narrow tube leading from a plastic bag of milk which hangs round the mother's neck. The tube is strapped to the breast and the baby sucks the nipple and tube together. Using this method adoptive parents have managed to establish full breast feeding of their single babies. Although no case has yet been reported there is no reason why adopted twins should not be breast fed in this way.

There have been occasional reports of a mother who has given one of her babies to another lactating mother to feed (Mead 1957).

BOTTLE-FEEDING

The obvious advantage of bottle-feeding twins is that the task can be shared. In particular the father is able to play a larger role in the care of his babies.

The disadvantages include the increased cost, the greater amount of work in sterilizing bottles, making up feeds etc. and, most important, the inability to nurse and feed both babies simultaneously. It is possible to nurse one baby by propping the other in a cushion but many mothers resort to propping both. This means that the babies have no direct contact with the mother. A few ingenious mothers devise ways of nursing one baby in their crossed legs and the other in their arms.

Many mothers are tempted to leave one or both babies feeding unattended (for example with the bottle supported by a cushion). The consequent dangers of choking should be obvious but may not always be to a harassed mother.

Preparation of the Feeds

Any safe short-cuts to this time-consuming chore should be welcomed. One of these is of course to make up the whole 24 hours' milk supply at the same time. A large plastic bucket or small dustbin will allow all bottles, jugs and teats to be sterilized together. The milk can be made up in large jugs but it should be transferred immediately to the bottles and refrigerated. If left in jugs and not thoroughly stirred at each serving the first feeds will be too dilute and the later ones dangerously concentrated (Twins Clubs Association 1981).

WEANING

If mother and babies are content there is no hurry for the babies to be weaned from the breast. Extended breast feeding is particularly valuable for twins as it ensures a continuing physical closeness with the mother. Ideally the twins should wean in their own time. One may well choose to do so several weeks before the other.

SOLID FOODS

Introducing solids to twin babies is an added chore for the already busy mother. It is therefore wise to postpone this as long as possible. There is rarely need to consider solids before 4 months of age. Even then one baby may well be ready to start before the other.

In the same way the children will have different tastes and appetites and these should be respected. Because one child asks for a drink or a snack it should not automatically be assumed that the other wants or needs the same.

Many mothers start with the firm intention of having a separate spoon and dish for each baby. Few keep it. When feeding them together it is much easier to use the same spoon and dish. Dishes, divided into two by a partition, are useful for gauging the approximate quantity eaten by each child.

Many twins are slow in learning to feed themselves as they lack opportunity. Mothers fear the mess and find it quicker to feed the children themselves. In extreme cases healthy twins may approach their second birthday with little idea of how to use a spoon (personal observation). This practice should be strongly discouraged. Exploration with food and the process of feeding is an important part of a child's development and should not be suppressed. Two high chairs, two large plastic bibs and an extremely large plastic mat are essential equipment and the children should then be given freedom to experiment.

9. The First Year

To be the mother of twins is the dream of many pregnant women. And for those 'doubly blessed' the happy expectations are reinforced by society's attitude which sees only the positive aspects of having twins. Few mothers are 'allowed' to think of the possible difficulties (Leonard 1959)—the difficulties of looking after two babies each of whom is likely to be more frail, more difficult to feed and more vulnerable to infection than the average single baby. And then there are the difficulties of responding to two babies, and perhaps hardest of all, of developing a relationship with two babies at the same time. Few mothers are prepared for these problems. Many therefore suffer painful shattering of happy expectations (Bryan 1977b).

Inevitably, a mother of twins spends less time with each baby than she would had she only one. This was clearly shown in Goshen-Gottstein's (1980) study from Israel of mothers of young twins in their homes. She found that mothers of twins spent 35–37% of their time on activities related to the twins whereas a mother with one baby spent as much as 22–29% of her time on that one baby.

Many mothers find that their reserves of both physical and emotional energy are expended before the end of each day, let alone the end of the first year. Many feel guilty that their previous domestic standards have not been upheld, that they are able to give so little attention to their husband. Marriages are often put under great strain during this time. Mothers deeply regret that they have so little time just to nurse and enjoy each baby (Bryan 1977b). This frustration of the need to identify with one baby is particularly keenly felt by those mothers for whom the twins are their firstborn children. This is partly because the normal caretaking activities are bound to take longer in inexperienced hands, but also because the mother feels cheated of a unique relationship. The main reason many mothers want a third (single) child is to have the experience of which they have been deprived—that of giving their undivided attention and love to one baby (Leonard 1959).

Over the last few years there has been increasing concern about the prevalence of depression amongst mothers of young children. Incidences as high as 40% have been reported amongst working-class mothers at home with young children (Wolkind 1981). The most important precipitating factors are stress and social isolation. Mothers of twins are thus especially vulnerable. Yet surprisingly there is little reference to mothers of twins in studies of postnatal depression.

The only study is a recent one by Powell (1981) who showed that mothers of firstborn twins suffered significantly more from atypical depression than mothers of singleton controls. This form of depression is characterized more by anxiety-related symptoms and the mothers were more irritable and tearful and had more feelings of self-criticism.

But many of these symptoms are also those associated with fatigue. Most mothers of young twins are of course often extremely tired. Whether true depression is more prevalent amongst these mothers has not been established. It is not impossible that true depression is less common amongst them than amongst mothers with single children for the very reason that two babies gives them a legitimate excuse for feeling so harassed and exhausted.

MANAGEMENT

Any saving of energy by reducing the physical burden of twins makes a mother better able to face the inevitable emotional strain. Too many mothers could have saved many exhausting hours had they been given more advice on the practical care of two babies and perhaps had they been readier to accept outside help (Bryan 1977*b*). Too many learn by trial and error although parents from, for instance, the local twins club could have given useful guidance.

Many mothers are too proud to accept help with domestic chores and continue doing these whilst allowing friends, for instance, to feed the babies. It needs emphasizing that offers of help should usually be diverted to other tasks so that the mother can spend more time with the babies.

There will, of course, be times when the mother welcomes a break from her babies. Indeed her mothering may be enhanced by the feeling that she can escape from that role occasionally and give space to her own needs.

Practical aspects of feeding have been discussed in Chapter 8. Washing (and drying) is also time consuming and fuss-free clothes are invaluable. Those needing ironing should be avoided. A tumble dryer is money well spent, for those who can afford one, and reduces the number of nappies needed. Mothers often struggle to bath their babies daily, believing this vital to health. There is plainly no need for this and most cannot easily bath two babies without a second pair of hands. It may well be advisable to limit bathing to times when father's help is available or otherwise to bath each separately on alternate days.

Many mothers complain of the isolation they feel during the first year. In a group of London mothers Clegg (1982, personal communication) found that one of the commonest complaints was of immobility leading to isolation. Mothers saw less of their friends and therefore got little feedback on how well they were coping and little encouragement. They felt out of touch with their former life and had little chance of outside entertainment. Their husbands often had to take time off work (and often used up their remaining annual leave) to accompany them, for instance, to the clinic or hospital appointment. Because they are confined to home or the immediate vicinity, mothers become increasingly reliant on their husbands; which can reduce their self-esteem or strain the marriage.

Those who would have taken one baby and visited friends regularly often find the performance of getting two babies ready, getting them there and then anxiously keeping an eye on two crawlers in someone else's precious home is not worth the strain. The majority lack a car in the daytime and for them transport is a major problem. Public transport with two babies in arms (plus pushchair and shopping) is almost impossible. In one group of 23 mothers only one took a bus alone with the twins during the first year. And she returned by taxi!

One bold mother took twins and an older brother on a tricycle. Most stick to their feet with a twin pram, pushchair or buggy. Two single buggies clipped together have the advantage that they can be separated at weekends or at other times when a second pair of hands is available. Likewise a single buggy can be clipped onto a twin buggy if three children need transporting. Sometimes a mother prefers to have one baby in a sling and the other in a pushchair. Some may carry both in slings one in front and one on her back.

Sleep

The survival of a mother, let alone the happiness of the family, can ultimately depend on whether or not the twins allow the family a good night's sleep. One wakeful baby can be disruptive enough.

There is obviously no simple answer to sleep problems nor a single arrangement that suits every family. The number of rooms available, their ambient temperature and the sleeping patterns of the babies all have to be considered. However many parents have blamed themselves in retrospect for allowing unnecessarily troublesome sleep patterns to develop in their twins.

During the early months a cot divided by a partition so that one baby sleeps at either end is satisfactory. Later, when they are in separate cots, some babies are comforted by being close enough to touch each other. If they do wake they may then resettle on their own. On the other hand many disturb each other so that if one wakes the second is woken unnecessarily. The cots should then be well separated and when practicable, perhaps even put in different rooms.

Mothers may actually reinforce bad sleeping habits. For instance a mother may rush, at the first whimper, to comfort one so as to prevent the other being disturbed. The children may welcome this easily won attention and demand it more and more. If sleeping separately the wakeful child may be left longer and a vicious circle may be avoided.

It is often assumed that if there are several children in the family the twins should always sleep together. However some families find that it is much better to separate the twins, each or one sleeping with another sibling.

FATHER'S ROLE

Clearly a mother with twins will turn to her partner for help very much more than she would do for a single child. Most fathers seem to respond well to this call (Bryan 1977*b*). The father's role has changed greatly in the last 10 or 20 years. They were already involved in many domestic tasks and the social climate now encourages them to take a more active part in the care of the children. Economic circumstances have pointed in the same direction. Women are sometimes now the main wage earners and with the additional expenses it may be essential for a mother of twins to continue earning. Thus in some families the father may be responsible for a substantial amount of the twins' care.

Although twins tend to have less contact than singletons with both their mother and their father the proportionate amount of time spent with their father is likely to be greater. It is not surprising therefore that Lytton (1980) found that more 2-year-old boy twins than singletons chose their father as their primary figures of attachment. This is one of the few bonuses for the father.

Nevertheless he may find the first year, in particular, a severe strain. He is almost bound to lose some of his wife's attention and care. He may become jealous of the demanding twins. Because of the added financial strain of a larger family he may also have to work longer hours, or more likely, cut down on luxuries. On top of all this he is then expected, and rightly, to help with the children and domestic tasks to an entirely unaccustomed degree. Because of all this the position and feelings of fathers of twins deserves more attention than they often receive and contact made possible through the Twins Clubs Association can be valuable.

IDENTIFICATION

Despite increasing awareness of the importance of twins being encouraged to develop their own individuality from the start, many parents find it difficult in practice during the first year. Social pressures and attitudes militate against it. Friends, relatives and particularly grandparents want to celebrate twins and like to see the children dressed alike. Few take the trouble to call the babies by their names. Indeed many parents fail to do so. In the case of MZ twins some even forget which name they originally gave to each child. Zazzo (1960) found that 10% of the parents of MZ twins did not remember their original naming.

And yet patterns set in the first year are difficult to change. Many parents, both for simplicity and for their own satisfaction, initially dress the babies alike with the firm intention of changing ater. But then the babies get used to looking alike and resent a change. Many parents who leave the change until the second or third year meet with vehement opposition. One pair as young as 10 months old when given different clothes for the first time refused to be consoled until they were allowed to be dressed alike again.

Obviously clothes should not be the only way of recognizing a child and any distinctive feature should be pointed out to friends. There may be a place for initialled or discretely named clothes for MZ twins and people should then be encouraged to use the names.

Photography is another context in which parents tend to treat their children as a unit. Quite often a family has no photographs of either child on his own. Worse still, parents sometimes cannot remember who is who. A note should be made each time. Twins are even more difficult to distinguish in photographs than real life. A poignant example arose with two-and-a-half-year-old MZ boys. The children had been photographed many times but always together. One twin suddenly died of meningitis. The father, in particular, could not bear to see photographs of the dead son. This meant that all pictures of the survivor were hidden away.

INTRAPAIR RELATIONSHIPS

From the start the emotional environment of a twin baby differs radically from that of a singleton for he must develop two strong emotional ties simultaneously; to the mother and to the co-twin. His most constant companion is his twin rather than his mother. And he is likely to be further confused by many changes of caretaker. Not only will the father handle the babies more but others including relatives and neighbours are more likely to be involved in caretaking activities, particularly feeding.

The age at which twins seem to become distinctly aware of each other varies greatly but certainly by 5 or 6 months they are sufficiently comforted by each other's presence for it to have a quieting effect (Leonard 1959). Too often parents, busy with household chores, take advantage of this fact, and assume that mother's attention is less necessary.

At this age, when most babies are beginning to explore their own bodies, twins may spend as much time in discovering that of their twin. Indeed, initially they make no distinction. It is not uncommon to see twins peacefully sucking each other's thumbs. It may be painful stimuli such as a bite of the other's finger that give the first indications to an infant of the limits of his own body image.

MATERNAL ATTITUDES

Most mothers want to treat their twin babies equally and plan to give them the same amount of time and attention. In practice this is not easy as one baby, often the smaller, can be much more demanding. Few mothers can give their full attention to a placid, seemingly contented, baby whilst the other baby is crying. Too often she is unable to concentrate fully on either baby. For instance she may be feeding one whilst soothing the other.

It is likely that the physical similarity of the babies, particularly of MZ twins, can be a barrier to the formation of a close relationship. Difficulty in distinguishing her babies must inhibit a mother's bonding.

The mother's attitude to the smaller of a pair varies. She may reject it with the feeling that it is in some way imperfect. The rejection may be promoted by inadequate bonding in the neonatal period (see p.97). On the other hand its very smallness and weakness may inspire special care and protection. Several studies have shown the latter reaction to be the more common, at least during the first year (Allen et al. 1971; 1976). This extra attention to the weaker baby may to some extent compensate for its initial deficit and facilitate its development in relation to its co-twin (Field and Widmayer 1980).

Some parents have unjustifiably higher expectations of the larger twin, even if the smaller one has been fit and well from the start. They assume for instance, that the larger one will walk first and expect other skills, even those unrelated to strength such as speech, to be more advanced (personal observation).

SIBLINGS

The effect of twins on other siblings has attracted little attention yet many of these children are deeply affected, even damaged, by the presence of an inseparable pair within the family. This is particularly so where there is only one single child: he may feel very isolated. His parents are a pair, so are the twins. Both seem to exclude him and very often the twins do. The isolation is intensified if the twins have their own language or other communication.

Bernstein (1980) goes as far as to say that older siblings may feel incomplete and 'search' for their own twin using doll or animal substitutes. They may have a special fear of being alone, particularly at nights. The toddler who has been used to the relatively straightforward relationship with two parents may be agonizingly confused by the sudden influx not only of twins but of the many new relationships they bring about.

He is deprived of much of his mother's time and attention. She, at least, may be aware of the problem; not so the many well meaning but thoughtless friends and acquaintances who focus all attention and admiration on the twins and do not see the unhappiness of the older child (Fig. 9.1). One mother was so concerned by this phenomenon that she had a seat especially arranged on the pushchair pram so that the twins could not be seen until the toddler had been acknowledged.

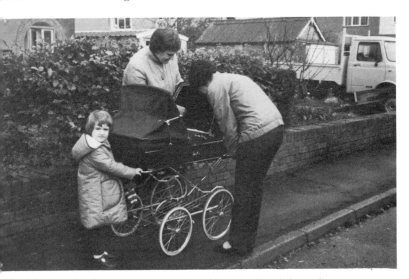

Fig. 9.1. Attention focussed on young twins while elder sister is ignored.

Single children, especially those close in age to the twins, may need more help and support than the twins themselves. This is rarely appreciated and we need to learn more about this neglected group.

On the whole the twins themselves benefit from having siblings. The more there are the looser their own bond is likely to become. In this respect DZ twins have some advantage over MZ in that they tend to come from larger families (Phillips and Watkinson 1981).

SUDDEN INFANT DEATH SYNDROME

The sudden unexpected death of an infant during the first year is a tragedy which can hit any family. Some infants however are known to be at particular risk and twins are amongst these. The incidence of the 'sudden infant death syndrome' (SIDS) or 'cot death' appears to be about twice that of infants in general (Carpenter 1965; Kraus and Borhani 1972). Amongst triplets the risk is higher still (Kraus and Borhani 1972). Like- and unlike-sexed pairs appear to be equally affected, as do both males and females (Carpenter 1965; Froggatt et al. 1971).

SIDS is known to be more common amongst prematurely born infants and those who have been separated from their mothers at birth. Thus it is not surprising that twins are more vulnerable. However, it would seem that the twinship in itself adds a further risk factor and the reason for this is not clear (Carpenter et al. 1979).

In families where one infant has died unexpectedly subsequent children have a five- to tenfold greater risk of themselves dying unexpectedly (Carpenter et al. 1979). Amongst twins the risk is higher still. There have now been many reports of both twins dying either at the same time or within a few days of each other (Cooke and Welch 1964; Carpenter 1965; Froggatt et al. 1971; Kraus and Borhani 1972). Occasionally both babies are found dead in the cot together.

One study found that the concordance rate for SIDS in like-sexed twins was 8.6% and in unlike 7.6% (Spiers 1974). In another series of 112 cases of SIDS in twins over half the co-twins had some abnormal signs around the time of the death of their twin and two died on the same day. On the other hand in 39% of pairs the parents had recognized no abnormal signs in either the dead twin or the survivor (Carpenter 1965). It appears that the excessive risk to the co-twin lasts only for 1 month and that much the most critical period is the first few days. For this reason some would advocate immediate and very close supervision of the surviving twin if not several days of observation in hospital (Emery 1979).

The effects on the family and, in particular, on the surviving twin of an unexpected death in infancy are discussed in Chapter 13.

10. The Preschool Twin

The preschool period is an especially critical time for twin children. It is important enough for singletons in that problems in those early years can have a lasting effect on their adult personality. In twin children however, the considerable extra complication is whether he will become properly independent or whether he must for ever function as half of a duo, unable to cope without the constant support of his co-twin.

INTRAPAIR RELATIONSHIP

Despite some inevitable sibling rivalries and jealousies, twins are usually strongly interdependent. They always have each other and therefore tend to be less dependent on others, not least their mother. Mothers often say that their twin children appear to have less need of parental approval and are less responsive to parental guidance and discipline.

When disappointed in their parents they turn to each other for consolation. Indeed this very interdependence and companionship may be vital to the emotional survival of some twins. Koluchova (1972) describes a pair of MZ boys who were isolated from the outside world from the age of 18 months to 7 years. They were deprived of any stimulation, spent many hours each day in the cellar and their only toys were a few bricks. They were frequently beaten by their stepmother. Their remarkable progress when removed from this environment and their apparent lack of long-term damage has been attributed to their close attachment to each other (Koluchova 1976; Editorial 1976).

Most twins do not seem to mind which of them was born first. Nor of course should they. Occasionally a firstborn boasts of his superiority. When this happens a parent might tell the story of the African tribe where the secondborn is considered senior. They say it is only after the firstborn has checked that the world is ready to receive him is the second twin delivered.

For a MZ twin the differentiation of his own ego and body from those of his partner must be a complicated process. If dressed alike the process may well be delayed still further. DZ twins learn to identify their mirror images several months before MZ twins (Burlingham 1952) and the majority of twins recognize the reflection of their co-twin in a mirror before their own (Bernabei and Levi 1976) (Fig. 10.1). The confusion was exemplified by the

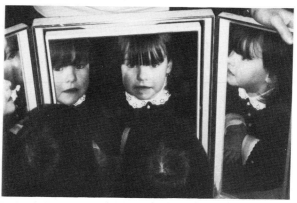

Fig. 10.1. MZ twins and their mirror images.

5-year-old MZ girl who when trying on a new dress told her twin to stand in front of her, 'So that I can see what I look like' (Mittler 1971).

Many twins respond to the name of the other twin as well as their own and often call themselves by their twin's name. For instance in a pair of MZ twins, Bert referred to his brother, Bill, as 'other-one-Bert' (Burlingham 1952). Leonard (1959) found that 60% of 2-year-old single children gave their own name on request whereas only 40% of twins did so.

BEHAVIOUR

Personality differences in twins are often apparent from a very early age. These are often shown first in differing feeding patterns. One baby may attack the teat or nipple with gusto and gulp the whole feed down in a few minutes whereas the other may choose to take it slowly over half an hour with breaks to rest and look around. One may demand frequent small feeds. The other may remain content for many hours.

Matheny and Brown (1971) found that birth order was not an important influence on behaviour. Birth weight discordance, however, led to more differences. Of 18 weight-concordant pairs only two showed markedly discrepant behaviour whereas in ten out of 18 weight-discordant pairs behaviour significantly differed. The lighter twin tended to have more 'problem' behaviours and was less proficient in aspects of cognitive behaviour.

Gifford et al. (1966) vividly illustrate these points in describing the progress of a pair of birth-weight-discordant MZ girls from birth to 6 years. The larger was always the more contented, placid and serious whereas the smaller was more active, impetuous and charming. Their IQ scores at 4 years were almost identical but the children's approach to the test was entirely different.

In the Louisville Twin Study over 200 mothers were interviewed periodically about the behaviour of their twins. At 1 year the differences were mainly in temper and attention span whereas by 4 years the main difference was in the degree of sociability (Wilson et al. 1971).

Not surprisingly, there was a higher degree of concordance in behaviour between MZ twins than DZ. However this effect of zygosity does not necessarily apply equally to interests and activities. In young children, at least, it appears that their activities are more a result of parental influence than any particular personality trait. Lytton (1980) found that 2- to 3-year-old MZ boys were no more similar in their choice of toys or forms of play than DZ. Later however the pattern changes. By 6 years Loehlin and Nichols (1976) found a significantly greater similarity in the activities of MZ than DZ twins.

Twins should always be encouraged to develop their own interests. If one asks to go to a football match there is no reason to assume his brother will also want to. If one is tired or hungry, why should the other automatically be so?

Separate outings should be arranged from an early age. Not only do they increase the twin child's independence but most single children (and adults) find it easier to build relationships one-to-one than one-to-two.

Several workers have shown that there is no correlation between similarity of appearance and similarity of behaviour within a twin pair (Cohen et al. 1975; Matheny et al. 1976; Plomin et al. 1976) This is perhaps not surprising as the more alike two children appear the greater may be their need to differ in behaviour.

Wilson found a surprising degree of age-to-age stability in intrapair behavioural differences. But this is by no means invariable. Many mothers report a switching, particularly in leadership, from time to time. Which twin dominates may vary with the situation (Lytton 1980).

A group of children who were defined by their mothers as being the dominant of a pair of twins were compared with their co-twins. The main differentiating factor was that the dominant twin tended to talk more than his partner. There was no intrapair difference in their verbal IQ, in their size, or in their degree of parental attachment (Lytton 1980).

I have already suggested that the natural individuality of twins—as of all children—should be respected, indeed encouraged (see p.123). There is, however, a danger of some parents artificially accentuating differences of personality or behaviour. It is inevitable that parents should constantly compare and contrast the behaviours of two children of the same age. And indeed look for differences. But this process often leads to the exaggeration of character traits which in fact lie well within the normal range. Parents may therefore speak of the 'placid' or 'lively' one of their twins and relatives and friends soon learn these sterotypes and, perhaps unconsciously, respond to the two children accordingly. More serious, however, is the fact that children tend to live up to parental expectations of being the one who is 'good' or 'naughty', 'quiet' or 'noisy', 'untidy' or 'tidy'. Parents should be helped to realize both that a balance has to be struck between encouraging and exaggerating differences between their children and that the range of 'normal' behaviour is wide and that children vary greatly, for instance, in their sociability or in their degree of attentiveness.

Parents usually believe themselves to be equally fond of each twin but this is not necessarily shown in their behaviour towards them. One child may be blamed for more misdemeanors than he deserves whereas the same actions in the other may pass apparently unnoticed. If parents expect certain behaviour they tend only to notice when the expectation is fulfilled. Goshen-Gottstein (1980) describes a pair of twins whom the mother had 'labelled' as early as 7 months—Ruben, the boy, as naughty and wild and Ruby, the girl as sweet and easier. Regular observation of the children did not confirm these differences yet at the age of two the mother still treated them according to this pattern. She often wrongly suspected Ruben of aggression towards a baby brother but was blind to the several occasions on which Ruby pulled the baby's hair.

On the other hand some mothers do recognize that they feel closer to one baby than the other. They may feel unhappy and ashamed about these feelings: many do not admit to them until months or years later. Such mothers (or fathers) might have been greatly relieved to know at the time that these unequal affections are not unusual and that most resolve themselves over time.

Young twins may have greater difficulty with social interaction than singletons. Kim et al. (1969) found that 3½-year-old twins in a nursery were more solitary, less affectionate and less aggressive. This may well be due to the relative isolation of a twin unit because, by the age of 5½, after 2 years in the nursery, these twins had overcome their inhibitions and their behaviour was not significantly different from singletons of the same age.

LATERALITY

Over no aspect of twinning has there been more disagreement than over laterality. The reported frequency of left-handedness in twins has varied from 5% to as much as 31% and even the effect of zygosity is a source of contention. One study showed that left-handedness was three times more common in MZ than DZ twins. Another found the incidence in MZ twins to be half that of DZ. In only 11 out of 18 studies was left-handedness found to be more common amongst MZ twins (McManus 1980).

Many earlier studies suggested a higher incidence of left-handedness in twins. More recently these conclusions have been challenged (McManus 1980). McManus analysed 19 studies of laterality in twins and found that none of them were satisfactory. Criteria had varied and rarely were twins and singletons seen by the same investigators. Most of the studies had been made before the advent of reliable zygosity determinations and some had actually assumed that symmetry reversal was pathognomonic of monozygosity (Newman 1928).

Several workers agree with McManus that there is no significantly higher incidence of left-handedness amongst twins (Husén 1959; Zazzo 1960; Koch 1966). Phillips (1981b) points out that to use the writing hand as a measure of laterality may be misleading as this is subject to cultural pressures. In the Birmingham study he found that 86% of twin children had consistent laterality for writing and for manual skills and that 14% of these were left handed. Six per cent differed in the hand they used for writing from that used for manual skills. The remaining 14% had mixed laterality. This last group was nearly twice as large as that found amongst singletons. The overall incidence of left-handedness in twins was higher than that in singletons but significant only at the 10% level. However intrapair concordancy for left handedness was five times the expected figure.

There may well be two separate populations of left-handed children. One of these groups would be genetically determined and hence no more common amongst twins than singletons. The second 'pathological' group would be that of children whose left-handedness is a result of an insult to the normally dominant left cerebral hemisphere during the intrauterine or perinatal periods. This group is likely to be disproportionately represented amongst twins.

Mirror Imaging

It is often said that MZ twins can be mirror images of each other which means that they have lateral asymmetry including the reversal of superficial features such as birthmarks and hair whorls, the reversal of internal organs (situs inversus) and opposite handedness. It has been thought that this lateral asymmetry would arise from the late division of the embryo when the left and right sides have already been determined.

However there is no concrete evidence for the existence of mirror imaging in MZ twins and several authors have found that particular asymmetries in twins are no more common than could be expected by chance (Torgersen 1950; Husén 1959; Bulmer 1970). Furthermore the process and timing of embryonic differentiation is not in fact sufficiently understood for embryologists to establish the basis for a theory of lateral asymmetry (Corney and Robson 1975).

LANGUAGE

Since the 1930s it has been recognized that twins are slower in their language development than singletons (Day 1932; Davis 1937). Many twin children whose overall intelligence is normal show significant deficits in their verbal performance (Alm 1953). Alm found that, by 4 years, twin children were 6 months behind singletons and, by defining language delay as a failure to use a sentence at 30 months of age, Zazzo (1979) found that 64% of MZ and 43% of DZ twins were retarded.

In her study of 5- to 6-year-old firstborn North American boys Koch (1966) found that twins were less talkative than singletons. Watts and Lytton (1980) found that by 9 years the verbal performance of twin boys was still delayed.

The most comprehensive large study of speech development in twins was that by Mittler (1976). He studied 200 4-year-old twins—30% MZ and 70% DZ—and applied the Illinois Test of Psycholinguistic Abilities which includes subtests for nine different aspects of speech development. He found that twins had an overall score 6 months behind that of singletons and that performance was influenced neither by zygosity nor birth order. Twins performed less well than singletons in all except one subtest and the exception was for speed of reaction to speech. Perhaps the constant presence of another competing recipient for communications from parents stimulates the development of this particular skill.

Savič (1980) has studied the pattern of communication between twins and their mothers in detail. As a result of her close observation of three pairs of twins over a 2-year period from 1 to 3 years of age she concluded that twins pass through the stages of speech development in a different way to singletons. Twins have to develop a much more complicated form of interaction. They must learn earlier how to communicate within a triad and when to engage and disengage in discourse. Concentration on this essential skill may mean that other aspects of speech development are postponed.

A particularly interesting finding in Mittler's study was that of the much greater effect of social class on language development in singletons than twins. In singletons there were 12 points (53 *vs.* 41) difference in scores between social class I and II and social class IV and V whereas the difference between the same groups in twins was only five points (44 *vs.* 39). Possibly the twin situation is such that children are less able to take advantage of their linguistically favourable environment. It may well be that some mothers from social class I and II, who would normally have looked after a single child on their own, employ help (generally less educated than themselves) when there are two children.

However, even with twins, the education of the mother does to some degree affect the speech development of the children. Lytton and Conway (1977) found that at 2½ years MZ boys had significantly less good verbal skills than DZ and that this could be entirely accounted for by the difference in mothers' education between the two groups.

Speech delay in twins is neither inevitable nor irremediable and it has been well demonstrated that twins can make conspicuous progress with appropriate teaching (Koluchova 1972, 1976; Douglas and Sutton 1978). Mittler (1971) tells a remarkable story about 4-year-old twin boys. The mother sought help because the boys had no speech, were overactive and wild. She was at her wits' end. Assessment showed that their intellectual function was subnormal and they both had IQs in the low 60s. The mother was advised to treat and talk to them individually, to dress them differently and in every way to try to prevent them acting, or being thought of, as a single unit. One year later they were transformed. Their speech was fluent and an IQ assessment gave them each a score of 120. It is plainly vital that more is learnt about detrimental factors in the early environment of twins and remedial efforts are not delayed.

Earlier workers assumed that delay in speech development of twins was related to the perinatal hazards of a multiple birth. However, it is now apparent that differences in the postnatal environment must be largely responsible. The most tangible evidence of this is shown in the development of single surviving twins. These children have perinatal experiences similar to, if not worse than, members of surviving pairs but their postnatal environment is that of a singleton. These single surviving twins were found to perform significantly better than twins and almost as well as singletons in their verbal skills. The mean score for single survivors (98.8) was only 1.3 points below that of singletons (100.1) whereas the twins scored 95.7. The difference between singletons and single survivors was further reduced to 0.7 when adjustment was made for the maternal age and birth rank of twins (Record et al. 1970).

Although no single factor has been isolated as the cause of language handicap in twins recent workers, in particular Lytton and his colleagues in Canada, have shed much light on the differences between the environment in which a twin is brought up and that of a singleton. Many of these differences could be expected to militate against optimal language development. It has also been suggested that twins have less need to use the conventional form of communication, language, as they have so many other means of relating to each other (Zazzo 1960).

From the very start twins face problems of communication. There is the almost constant presence of three potential participants in any act of communication, so there are always two recipients and two responders to any message within the triad.

Verbal interaction of all kinds appears to be reduced in families with twins. Not only do twins talk less than singletons but parents of twins communicate less with their children. When they do talk they tend to use shorter and grammatically less complex utterances (Lytton and Conway 1977). This may in part be because the mother has less time and more strain but many mothers also mistakenly believe that twins have less need of maternal attention because they entertain or comfort each other.

Mothers are less responsive to the distress or demands of twin children. They also give fewer commands, suggestions and, in particular, explanations. Rules are less consistently carried through. Mothers also demonstrate less affectionate behaviour and give less praise and approval (Lytton 1980).

Acquisition of speech is a highly complex process which is heavily dependent on personal interaction. Children learn to speak through learning, imitation and stimulation. The main models for singletons are parents or older siblings. For the twin the main

Table 10.1. Communication between 1- to 3-year-old twins and their mother (Savič 1980)

Direction of communication	% Time
Mother ⇄ Twin	20.33
Twin ⇄ Mother	18.41
Twin ⇄ Twin	13.88
Twin ⟶ Mother	29.65
Mother ⟶ Twin	0.91
Non-directed	9.73
Triadic	6.49

model is the co-twin. Thus speech is likely to be immature and deviations from normal will be reinforced. Some observers have gone so far as to assume that twins communicate with each other in preference to their mother. Savič (1980) found that this was not so. Twins are often forced into communicating mainly with each other but given the choice they prefer relating to their mother. In addressing the adult they will more often choose the diadic than triadic forms of communication (see Table 10.1). In a detailed study of communication in three pairs of twins Savič found that twin children directed speech to their mother over twice as often as to their co-twin.

Single mothers of twins appear to compensate for the absence of the father by providing sterner discipline and criticism. Although they reassured their children even less than married mothers of twins they gave them greater stimulation and these children tended to have greater verbal comprehension than other twins (Lytton 1980). These findings are the results of a study of only five families so no firm conclusions can be drawn. Nevertheless it does show that compensation for the lack of a second parent can be made in at least some aspects of development.

Cryptophasia

Much has been made of the 'secret language' of twins. There is no doubt that this cryptophasia or autonomous speech, a language quite incomprehensible to others, does exist. Occasional instances of isolated pairs with exclusive cryptophasia have been reported. Scobie (1979) described a pair of MZ girls who had little contact with anyone but each other during the first 5 years. They had developed their own relatively elaborate language. To others they had no recognizable language at all.

Exclusive cryptophasia is, however, extremely rare and there is little evidence that the use of this intertwin communication is in itself harmful to normal speech development. Incidences of about 40% amongst twins have been reported by several workers (Mittler 1970). Some have found cryptophasia to be more common amongst MZ twins (Alm 1953; Zazzo 1979). Zazzo (1979) considered that 48% of the 2½-year-old MZ twins he examined had cryptophasia and only 27% of DZ. Others have found no difference in the incidence in MZ and DZ twins.

Stuttering

Stuttering has been little studied in twins. Koch (1966) found that 11% of twins stuttered at one stage but only 6% were still doing so by the time they started school. The problem was more common amongst boy twins than girls. Rife (1940) found a slightly higher incidence amongst twins than singletons and like Koch (1966) found it to be equally common among MZ and DZ. Concordance, although low in both groups, was over twice as common amongst MZ twins.

ILLNESS IN TWINS

Apart from a vulnerability to infections in the early months due to prematurity, twins are, in general, neither more nor less prone to most physical illnesses than singletons. Malignant disease may however be an exception. It appears that some cancers may be less common in twin children. Hewitt and Stewart (1970) found that there were fewer cases of non-radiogenic cancers than would be expected amongst like-sexed twins who died before their tenth birthday and they suggested that this was due to the elimination of those fetuses whose later neoplasms would have resulted from cell damage incurred at, or shortly after, conception.

Twins under school age also appear to be less prone to leukaemia, which is surprising as twins are, if anything, more likely to be exposed to radiation in intrauterine life. Leukaemia, when it does occur, was found to be more common in pairs of disparate birth weight. The larger infant is the one more commonly affected (Jackson et al. 1969).

Staying in Hospital

If one twin has to go into hospital during the early years the effect on both children may be shattering. Not only are they separated from each other, often for the first time, but one or other will be separated from his mother too. If the admission is unexpected there will not even be chance to prepare the children for separation. Yet many hospitals will not allow admission to the healthy twin and few actually recommend it. In one study of 139 twins admitted to hospital before the age of 7 years only one was accompanied by his twin for non-medical reasons (Griffiths 1981).

Thus every effort should be made to admit both children and the mother. In the rare instances where this is impossible then the healthy child should at least be allowed to stay with his twin throughout the day.

Accidents

No figures are available on the accident rate in twins but it would be surprising if it was not relatively high. It is often difficult to keep a simultaneous eye on two active crawlers or toddlers who have no sense of danger.

Worse than this however, is the terrifying daring of bold children encouraged by another. Siblings, let alone single children, rarely get into the same predicaments. In most pairs there is either an older child with some sense of reality or a younger one who is physically unable to tackle the project. With twins the combination of mutual encouragement and physical co-operation results in far more reckless feats—or attempts.

There is an added danger for MZ twins. If they are dressed alike particularly in outdoor clothes, many parents cannot distinguish

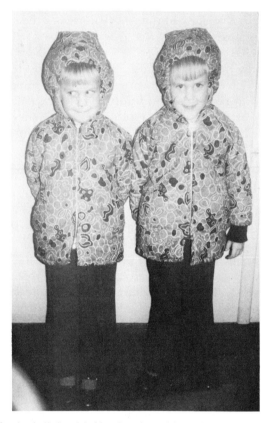

Fig. 10.2. MZ twins indistinguishable when dressed in outdoor clothes.

the two children at a distance. But if a child is about to chase a ball across a busy road a failure to call the correct name could cost a young life (Fig. 10.2).

Some children are undoubtedly accident prone but it is difficult to know whether an initial accident results in behaviour conducive to further disasters or whether such behaviour is inherent in particular children. Using twins from the Louisville Twin Study, Matheny et al. (1971) went some way to answering this question. They reviewed all pairs of twins in which at least one child had had an accident resulting in hospital admission. By referring to their previous records they found there were certain types of behaviour which were more common in the injured children than in their less accident-prone twins.

Child Abuse

The non-accidental injury (NAI) of a child by his parent is known to be more common in families under emotional or financial stress and amongst children who were premature or separated from their mother during the first days after birth. It would therefore be reasonable to expect that twins would be at exceptionally high risk of abuse. Accurate data on NAI in twins is difficult to find but there is, so far, no evidence to suggest an unduly high incidence amongst them.

On the NSPCC register of 'at risk' children, which covers 15% of the child population in the UK, the proportion of twins amongst those actually injured in 1977–78 was 2.4%—a figure little higher than the 2% of twins in the general population. The proportion classified as 'at risk' but not necessarily injured was a little higher (S. Creighton 1981, personal communication).

The reason why NAI is not even more common amongst twins is not immediately apparent. Possibly the fact that there is a second baby to whom a mother may divert her attention in moments of extreme exasperation with the other could prevent an attack at the crucial moment. It has also been suggested that a mother has lower expectations of twins and that this may act positively to prevent abuse. Twins are expected to be premature and therefore more difficult to manage. Mothers may feel less cheated of an easy, thriving contented baby if they had never expected one. They may therefore be more ready to accept a 'difficult' baby (A. Clegg 1981, personal communication). Nevertheless there are times when even the most caring mother may be tested to the edge of endurance and only with help and support may disaster then be avoided. The mother of DZ twin boys who were born at 28 weeks' gestation weighing 1 kg each was just such a case. At the age of 3 months after a very stormy neonatal period these much-wanted babies were finally taken home with much rejoicing to join their 18-month-old sister. They cried almost incessantly for the next 2 months, by which time the poor mother, despite the excellent support of her husband, was so exhausted and desperate that she begged not to be left alone as she feared that she might harm the babies. Fortunately she admitted to these feelings of aggression. She was given round-the-clock support and within a few months things were much better and the much-loved little boys have thrived. The mother has since given great understanding and support to other mothers living through similar crises.

Child abuse can, of course, take many forms. One of the most worrying forms that is often missed, is the so-called Munchausen syndrome by proxy (Meadow 1977). In these cases the mother creates symptoms and abnormalities in the child by various means including drugs and physical insults. This syndrome has been reported in a pair of MZ twins, who presented with recurrent unexplained bleeding (Lee 1979).

It is not uncommon for one child, particularly in pairs of different sex or size, to become the scapegoat and hence the target for aggression. If the situation becomes so serious that the abused child must be removed from his parents a dilemma arises. Must he also be separated from his twin or should his twin join him in Care and the second twin then be separated (unnecessarily) from his parents? There is no easy answer. But whatever happens the twins should continue to see as much of each other as possible.

11. Starting School

Starting school is an important milestone for any child. Both parents and children think about it a lot before the big day comes. When the children are twins there are many additional aspects to consider. The parents must decide whether the children should be in the same class, or even in the same school. Perhaps the twins should start together and be separated later. If so, at what stage?

There are no simple or universal answers to these questions and advantages and disadvantages will need to be weighed for each individual pair (Rowland 1981).

TOGETHER OR APART?

The normal stages of a child's development include the gradual loosening of the bond with his parents. Starting school is an important stage in this process. Twins have a second, often equally strong, bond to loosen—that with their co-twin. Most parents expect their twin children to be in separate classes when they reach secondary school but many need guidance in deciding whether to separate them earlier. Indeed many teachers also need guidance (see below).

Advantages of Separation

When separated from his twin a child can more easily develop his own personality and abilities. No longer need he only be compared with his twin and nor will he be so likely to have particular personality traits emphasized just because they are different from his twin (see p.124).

Some twins like to perform exactly the same as each other and they may contrive to achieve similar results at school. The brighter child may therefore tend to underachieve whereas the slower may be put under undue stress to keep up. Other pairs are conscious of differing abilities, real or imagined, and accept the varying roles expected of them. Either way the children would be better separated.

Parents themselves may become unnecessarily anxious about the children's progress if they are in the same class and their differences are therefore readily seen. Children vary not only in their rates of progress but also in the timing of periods of acceleration and periods of assimilation. Parents may be worried by these differences in performance. Just because one child is racing through the reading books and the other is taking them more slowly, there is no reason to assume that the second is failing. These differences are much less obvious when the twins are in different classes.

Girls tend to develop faster in the early school years and this can be a problem in mixed-sex pairs. The girl often tends to 'mother' the boy which, at the time, he may be quite happy to accept, but in the long term it may harm his relationships with the other children, particularly the boys.

Some twins are very dependent on each other. Obviously some degree of mutual support, particularly in the early days, can be beneficial. However if the dependence is either so intense that it excludes other relationships, or is so unbalanced that one twin performs on behalf of both, then it must be harmful. It is not uncommon to find pairs of 5-year-old twins in which one answers all the time regardless of who is asked the question.

An extreme example of this was seen in a pair of MZ boy twins who had changed schools many times due to their father's frequent changes of post in the armed forces. They finally reached their first school medical examination at the age of 8 years. One twin had always been the leader and had answered all questions addressed to his brother as well as to himself. It was only then found that the retiring twin had a severe degree of hearing loss. This had never been noticed owing to the co-twin's constant intervention on his behalf.

Sometimes if one twin is obviously more talented in a particular direction the other will opt out completely. For instance, if one is a star cricketer and the other only average the second may not wish to play at all. Had they been in different classes or schools the second twin would probably have been happy to join in with the others. In this way the less talented twin may not allow himself the chance to develop fully in many kinds of school activities.

School gives the child, often for the first time, a part of life that is independent of his parents. Some of this life he may want to keep to himself and not necessarily share with the family. If one twin repeatedly reports all that has happened to the other (whether it be good or bad) the second may be distressed and he is being denied his important right to privacy.

Twins together can make a powerful unit. If they combine forces to be disruptive they can cause chaos in a class and are then better separated as also where one tends to distract the other. Many twins use their 'twinship' to confuse teachers and entertain other children. This is harmless fun in small doses but can become a destructive and attention-seeking habit. Phillips and Watkinson (1981) found that 24% of twins played tricks of identity with teachers.

Disadvantages of Separation

When kept together twins seem to have less problem settling into school than single children (Koch 1966; J. Stevenson 1982, personal communication). This is no doubt because they feel less vulnerable. Although they have lost their mother they still have the security of their twin.

Most people would agree that if the twins like being together then they should start school in the same class, at least for the first term. If twins are so dependent on each other that they pine and do not join in school activities when parted, there is no point in enforcing separation. Usually this problem arises only with twins who have had no previous experience of acting independently. In these cases separation must be planned as a very gradual process. For instance, the first stage may be for children to sit at different tables within the same class or at mealtimes and then gradually progress from there.

Timing of Separation

If twins start together the timing of the separation must be carefully planned. It is usually better if they separate when a change is due anyway. Otherwise one will remain in the same room with the same teacher and friends and the other may feel rejected as he sets off alone into the unknown.

Some schools may be flexible enough to allow the children to move whenever it seems in their best interests. Others may have a more rigid policy and insist that changes only take place at certain stages in the school or at the beginning of the academic year. It is important that parents should discover the policy of their particular school as it may influence their initial choice of school.

CHOICE OF SCHOOL

In the UK it seems that most twins go to the same school as each other. In the Birmingham Twin Study 199 pairs of twins of primary school age were at the same school. One child was at a special school (for the handicapped) and his twin was at the normal primary school. One pair only was separated from choice (Phillips and Watkinson 1981). In the same study 13% were in different classes by the age of 7 years but only 2% were separated at 5 years. In Koch's study of North American children she found that many more were separated, particularly amongst the boys. At the age of 6 years, half the boys were in different classes and just under a quarter of the girls (Koch 1966).

In rural areas there will probably be only one local school and this is unlikely to have more than one class per year. The children must necessarily remain together. In towns, where there are more primary schools and most of them will be larger, parents have a choice. It is important to find out the school's policy on twins. It is surprising how many have a rigid view, either insisting that twins remain together or, less commonly, that they are always separated. Secondary schools appear less sensitive to the needs of twins than primary schools (Stevenson 1982) and parents may have to emphasize the importance of respecting the individuality of each child.

Teachers' Attitudes

Many teachers welcome the arrival of twins and are eager to accept advice from the parents as how best to help them cope with their twinship in school. Others still have set (often false) ideas about twins. They expect them to be slower than other children, to look alike and to like being treated alike. Many teachers assume that they will not be able to tell the twins apart and therefore make little effort to do so; they see them as a pair with no distinguishing differences in personality. Some teachers however may be too keen to compare and contrast the behaviour and abilities of the twins. Striking the balance is never easy.

PREPARATION

Twins, like any children, need long and careful preparation for school. They need particular help in learning to be independent of each other and the more each has been used to doing things on his own the easier will the transition be. Some mothers find that it is helpful if each attends some playgroup or nursery sessions on his own. One mother sent the twins together for one morning and on another two mornings one or the other went alone, which increased their independence and allowed them each a period of the mother's individed attention.

If twins are used to being dressed alike it is important that they get used to looking different. Initially twins, particularly MZ, find this disconcerting and it is helpful if this phase can be worked through before they start school.

STARTING SCHOOL

For those in separate classes it is often helpful if a friend or relative can come to school with the mother until the children have settled. Otherwise a mother may feel torn if both children are tearful and needing her and she has to leave one comfortless.

For twins who are not used to being separated the first few weeks are bound to be stressful. The teachers should be made aware of this. They should ensure that the twins see each other at intervals through the day and, for instance, sit together at meals.

If the twins are in the same class it is important that the teacher and the other children should be able easily to tell who's who. In MZ twins different hairstyles are helpful and, of course, different clothes. Initials or decorative name badges can be useful until everyone is sure they can tell them apart. It may be necessary specifically to ask the teacher not to refer to them as 'the twins'.

Unfortunately it is not only the teachers' attitudes that may be misguided. The parents themselves may insist on the children looking alike. One teacher had this problem with a pair of

11-year-old MZ twin girls who neither she nor their class mates could tell apart. The twins always dressed alike. Their abilities however, were quite different. One was intelligent and confident and the other was shy and found school work difficult. The teacher's approach to each child should have been very different but she found the constant confusion of identity a severe handicap to her relationship with them. She asked the mother if they could have some form of identification even if it was only a coloured hair slide. The mother adamantly refused.

On the whole twin children are popular although they may be less gregarious (Koch 1966). They usually have no trouble in making friends. They are used to co-operative games and are usually better at these than individual activities. Phillips and Watkinson (1981) found that most twins made some separate friends; only one-third of 7-year-olds always shared the same friends. Occasionally one twin may be much more outgoing than the other and have a much larger circle of friends.

12. Growth and Development of Twins

From the moment of conception twins are at a disadvantage. The problems facing twins both in intrauterine life and in early childhood have been described in earlier chapters. But what of their long-term mental and physical development? Is this affected by these earlier problems, or indeed by the 'twin situation'?

PHYSICAL GROWTH

In view of the relatively high proportion of twins who suffer from intrauterine growth retardation it is not surprising to find that on the average adult twins are smaller than singletons. Male twins in Sweden, at the time of their 'call-up' for military service, were 1.3 cm smaller than their singleton counterparts (Husén 1959). Perhaps more surprising is the relatively small discrepancy in adulthood considering the marked difference in size between twins and singletons at birth (see p.88). Several studies have shown a remarkable catch-up, particularly in the case of the smaller of a size-discrepant pair, during the first year (see below).

The most comprehensive data on growth in twins have come from the Louisville Twin Study in which 900 white North American twins were studied from birth. By 1979 over 400 had been followed beyond their eighth birthday and as a result Wilson (1979) has produced the centile charts for height, weight and occipitofrontal circumference shown in Figs. 12.1 and 12.2.

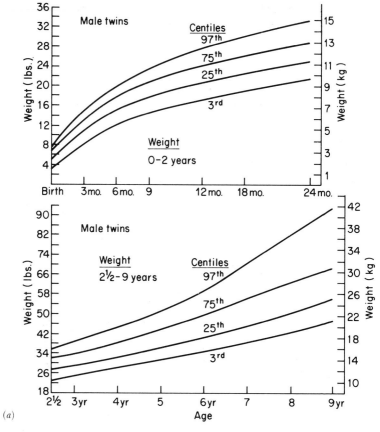

Fig. 12.1. Centile charts for weight in twins from 0 to 9 years. (a) Boys. (b) Girls.

By 4 years twins had almost caught up with singletons in height but less so in weight. Wilson suggests that this may be because the normal rate of replication of adipose cells during fetal life was reduced owing to the greater nutritional demands imposed by a twin pregnancy. On the other hand Chamberlain and Simpson (1977), in a random sample of nearly 200 British 3½-year-old twins, found that the twins were similarly proportioned to single-tons but were significantly lighter and shorter.

Wilson (1974a) found that the boys grew relatively faster during the first 6 months whereas the size of the girls accelerated during the third year. The catch-up of both sexes in relation to singletons continued and by 8 years of age there were no significant differ-ences in either height or weight between twins and singletons.

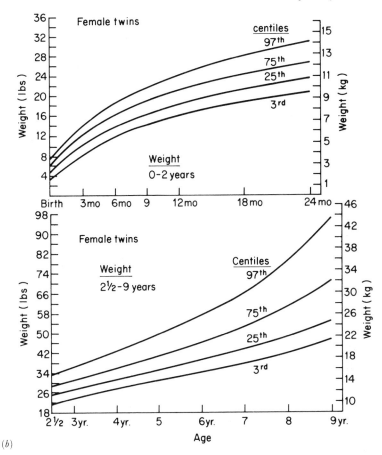

(b)

In the Louisville Study growth rates have not been shown in relation to birth weight. It may well be that larger pairs do better than smaller. Drillien (1964) found that, even with good home conditions, twins who weighed less than 2.5 kg at birth never made up their initial growth deficit. But a contemporary study is needed to confirm this point as the children in Drillien's study were born during an era when it was the practice to restrict the food intake of low birthweight babies.

A longitudinal study of growth patterns in older twins has been reported by Ljung et al. (1977). They followed over 300 twin pairs from 10 to 18 years. In boys they found that the differences in height, weight and peak growth velocity between twins and singletons were all small and much less than the differences between twin and singleton girls. The girls showed a significant

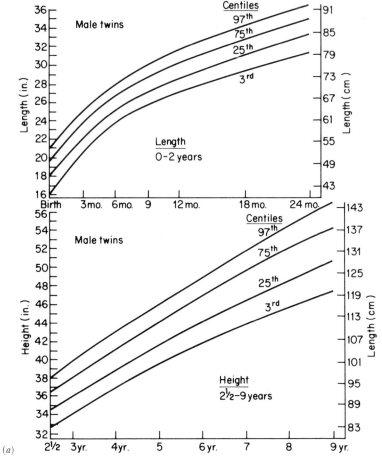

Fig. 12.2. Centile charts for height in twins from 0 to 9 years. (a) Boys. (b) Girls. From Wilson (1979) by permission of the author and the editors of *Annals of Human Biology*.

deficit particularly during puberty—their peak height velocity, peak weight velocity and menarche all came later than in singleton girls. It was suggested that this relatively better performance by twin boys might be due to selective survival as there is a higher early mortality amongst twin boys than twin girls (Figs. 12.3 and 12.4).

Zygosity

Over the years the growth of MZ twins becomes progressively more concordant and that of DZ less concordant (Wilson 1979). This is

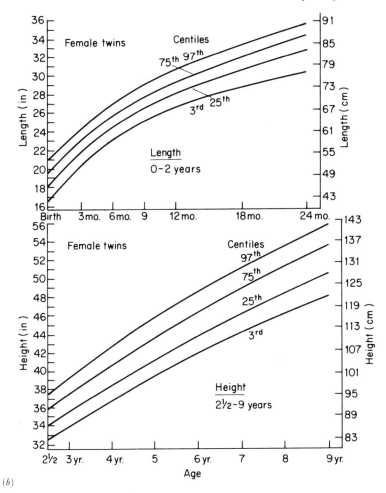

(b)

to be expected. As extrauterine environmental influences are likely to be similar for both members of a twin pair then the genetic influences will dictate any differences in growth pattern from birth onwards. In intrauterine life, however, the environment of one fetus may be very different from that of his co-twin, particularly in MZ pairs.

Genetic influences take time to counteract the effects of prenatal experience and it may be several years before long-term growth patterns are established. Tanner et al. (1956) showed that the 'genetic target curve' in singletons is not reached until the age of 2 or 3 years. Vandenberg and Falkner (1966) found the same

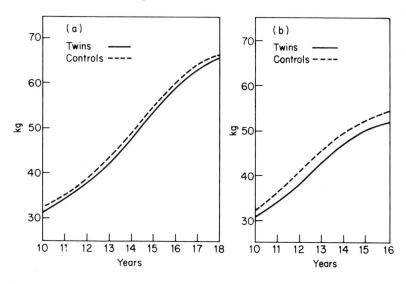

Fig. 12.3. Weight charts in twins 10–18 years compared with singletons. (a) Boys. (b) Girls. From Ljung et al. (1977) by permission of the authors and editors of *Annals of Human Biology.*

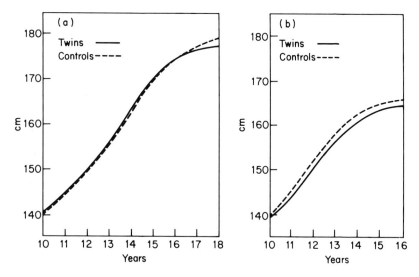

Fig. 12.4. Height charts in twins 10–18 years compared with singletons. (a) Boys. (b) Girls. From Ljung et al. (1977) by permission of the authors and editors of *Annals of Human Biology.*

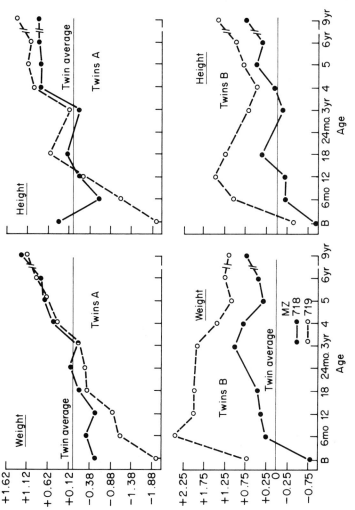

Fig. 12.5. Growth charts in two pairs of MZ twins of discrepant birth weight showing later similarity of intrapair growth. From Wilson (1979) by permission of the author and editors of *Annals of Human Biology*.

tendency in twins. The concordance for growth was very similar for MZ and like-sexed DZ twins during the first few months but thereafter the DZ twins became increasingly discordant. Not surprisingly, as they are dictated to by the same 'gene-action system', MZ twins tend also to have similar patterns of growth, coinciding their periods of growth spurt or latency (Fig. 12.5).

The effect of other intrauterine influences was considered by Falkner (1978). He found that postnatal growth in MZ twins can depend in part on types of placentation. MZ monochorionic pairs became progressively more similar in weight between birth and 4 years, their initial intrapair difference of 14.4% falling over the period to 2.9% whereas MZ dichorionic pairs maintained a remarkably similar intrapair discrepancy (9.5–10.7%) throughout.

Although intrapair comparisons of growth have been made in relation to zygosity most studies have not distinguished between MZ and DZ twins in comparing twins with singletons. It is possible that MZ twins have a reduced growth potential due to their loss of size in early embryonic life. This early zygote division has been proposed as an explanation for the lower birth weight of MZ twins (see p.42). Husén (1959) did find that adult male DZ twins were significantly (even if only 0.85 cm) taller than MZ twins. However genetic factors could also explain the DZ twins' greater height. Mothers of DZ twins are on average taller than MZ (see p.20).

Intrapair Discrepancies in Birth Weight

There is disagreement in the literature as to how the smaller of a pair of twins fares in the long term both physically and mentally.

Several workers have found that when there were large intrapair differences in birth weight in MZ twins then some discrepancy persists (Babson and Phillips 1973; Wilson 1979). In a group of ten MZ pairs with intrapair weight differences of over 750 g Wilson (1979) found that, at 6 years, the smaller twin was still significantly lighter, marginally shorter but had no significant reduction in IQ. There have, however, been several case reports of astonishing catch-ups (Buckler and Robinson 1974; Falkner 1978). One MZ twin, the donor in a fetofetal transfusion syndrome (see p.46), weighed 1560 g and his co-twin weighed 2700 g. By 18 months there was only 180 g difference in weight and by their ninth birthday the smaller was actually 1 cm taller than his brother.

Why some smaller MZ twins should show such a remarkable ability to catch up whilst others remain permanently smaller is uncertain. It may well be that there are two distinct groups of intrauterine growth-retarded twins. One, the catchers up, would be those who probably suffered from malnutrition only in the latter part of pregnancy and thus they had acquired their full cellular complement and, therefore, potential for growth. The other—the laggards—would be those whose differential growth was established early in pregnancy, thereby reducing their long-term growth potential.

MENTAL DEVELOPMENT

It is popularly said that twins are less clever than single children and many parents worry that this reduced intelligence will be a serious handicap to their children. It is true that most, although not all, studies have shown that the mean intelligence quotient (IQ) of twins is somewhat lower than that of singletons (Mehrotra and Maxwell 1949; Scottish Council for Research in Education 1953; Husén 1961; Drillien 1964; Record et al. 1970; Kranitz and Welcher 1971; Churchill and Henderson 1974; Myrianthopoulos et al. 1976; Zazzo 1979). However, the great majority of twins will be well within the normal range for singletons. Indeed there have been many examples of brilliant pairs of twins as well as individual twins in all walks of life (Scheinfeld 1973).

Husén (1961, 1963) reported a large study of Danish school-age twins of 11–15 years. He found that the mean IQ of twins was between ¼ and ⅓ standard deviation below that of singletons. This was not just due to a large number of low scorers. The overall distribution of scores was similar to that found in singletons but with the curve shifted to the left. Zazzo (1979) found that this was true throughout the socioeconomic groups, suggesting that even in the most favourable conditions twins were at a disadvantage.

Drillien (1964) found that at all ages between 6 months and 4 years the developmental quotients (DQ) of twins were lower than singletons. She divided both her singletons and twins into four groups according to birth weight. There was a positive correlation between birth weight and DQ in both twins and singletons at all ages, and twins scored consistently lower than singletons.

In the Louisville Study, however, it was found that although twins were relatively retarded at 18 months, they had caught up by their sixth birthday and by this age there was no significant difference between twins and singletons (Wilson 1974*b*). There is plainly scope for more research in this area. In considering the inferior performance of twins the detrimental effect of close sibling spacing in itself must not be forgotten. Singletons born close together are known to be at a disadvantage and twinship is the extreme example of close spacing. Zazzo (1960) demonstrated this. Whereas singletons in general scored 7 points higher in IQ testing than twins, siblings born close together were superior to twins by only 2.25 points.

Zygosity

Again, few studies have differentiated between MZ and DZ but where they do MZ twins are more alike in their mental development than DZ (Husén 1963; Wilson 1974*b*). MZ become increasingly concordant with age and parallel each other for spurts and lags (Fig. 12.6). DZ twins become progressively less concordant eventually matching singleton siblings as closely as they do each other (Wilson 1978, 1981).

Placentation

It has been suggested that differences in placentation might in themselves affect the long-term development of twins. Melnick and Myrianthopoulos (1979) did find significantly less variability in the intrapair scores of MZ monochorionic 7-year-old twins than MZ dichorionic. Indeed they found that intrapair differences in MZ dichorionic twins were surprisingly similar to those in DZ twins. It is difficult to explain this finding and others have not confirmed it (Brown 1977; Welch et al. 1978). If anything, MZ dichorionic twins could be expected to be more alike as they have smaller intrapair birth weight discrepancies and they are not at risk from the potentially long-term effects of the fetofetal transfusion syndrome.

Birth Weight

It is well known that small-for-dates singletons tend to have lower IQ scores than those who are appropriately grown at birth. It is not surprising, therefore, to find that within a pair of MZ twins the heavier born is likely to be more intelligent than his lighter co-twin (Scarr 1969; Munsinger 1977) and this applies throughout the socioeconomic groups (Willerman and Churchill 1967). Most

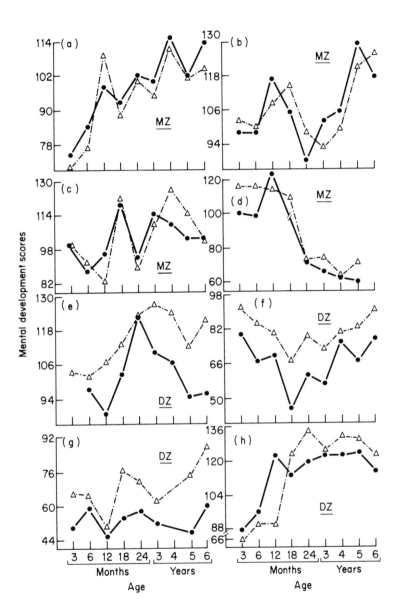

Fig. 12.6. Mental development of eight pairs of twins showing greater concordance in pattern in MZ pairs than in DZ. From Wilson (1978) by permission of the author and editors of *Science*. Copyright 1978 by the American Association for the Advancement of Science.

studies have shown this trend although some have not found that the difference reached levels of significance (Fujikura and Froehlich 1974).

Kaelber and Pugh (1969) compared a group of MZ twins who differed in birth weight by less than 300 g from their co-twin with a second whose intrapair discrepancies were over 300 g. The average IQ difference between the heavier and lighter twin in the first group was 0.48 whereas in the second it was 5.76. Scarr (1969) reported similar findings in a group of 52 MZ pairs.

Babson and Phillips (1973), in their serial observations of nine MZ pairs with an average birth weight difference of 36%, found that the lighter twin remained smaller and less intelligent into adulthood. However, there was less intrapair discrepancy in school performance than would have been expected from the results of the test scores, which suggests that the smaller twin had made an extra effort in order to compensate for his deficit.

Those who find that the smaller twin does less well blame the prenatal environment for his handicap whereas those who found that the little one does almost as well as his twin consider that the strength of the common genetic influence overrides other factors.

A common postnatal environment may blur the effects of birth weight discrepancies on mental development particularly if the smaller twin has the constant stimulus of a more intelligent twin and, probably, extra encouragement and help from parents. In order to eliminate these postnatal influences Munsinger (1977) studied 23 twins who were separated at birth and who appeared, from the literature, to have been of obviously differing size at birth. He surmised that in most cases, if not all, the fetofetal transfusion syndrome had been responsible for the differences. In this group the heavier twin had a higher IQ in 19 instances and the average discrepancy was 11.4 points, with an overall average IQ of 93.5. In contrast 26 pairs of separated twins of similar birth weight had a discrepancy of only 3.9 and an overall average IQ of 99.9. From these results he concluded that any estimates of heritability in behavioural genetics would be biased if MZ twins of discrepant birth weight were included and the strength of genetic influences would be underestimated.

HANDICAP IN TWINS

The parents of twins face not only the double risk of having a child with a handicap but because the children are twins the risk is further increased as many forms of handicap are more common amongst twins. The high incidence of congenital malformations has already been discussed (see p.48). Some twins who survive the dangers of the perinatal period are left with scars such as mental retardation or cerebral palsy. Others may be damaged as a direct result of their intrauterine twin relationship (see below).

Mental Retardation

It is generally agreed that mental retardation is more common in twins than singletons (Berg and Kirman 1960; Allen and Kallmann 1962). The only form that actually appears to be less common is that due to Trisomy 21—Down's syndrome.

Exact figures are difficult to obtain as much data are derived from institutionalized patients where there may be a selective bias. For instance a family might cope at home with one retarded child but be defeated by two. On the other hand if one of a pair of twins is handicapped the parents may feel less inclined to separate the two by sending one away. This also applies, of course, to other handicapping conditions such as cerebral palsy.

In studies of the general population severely handicapped individuals are often excluded, for instance in groups of schoolchildren or, in Husén's case, routine medical examinations for military enrolment. Nevertheless Husén (1959) found that the number of young adult twins with an IQ of less than 75 was twice that in the general population.

The secondborn twin and the smaller of a pair appear to be at greater risk than their co-twins (Berg and Kirman 1960), which would suggest that pre- and perinatal insults are the main aetiological factors. Likewise like-sexed or MZ twins are more commonly affected, probably due to their more hazardous intrauterine existence.

Cerebral Palsy

Many authors have found that twins are over-represented amongst children with cerebral palsy (Asher and Schonell 1950; Russell 1961; Eastman et al. 1962). Several have reported an incidence of over 7% amongst groups of cerebral palsied children (Benda 1952; Greenspan and Deaver 1953; Yue 1955), which is over three times the incidence of twin individuals in the general population. It seems that like-sexed twins are more likely to be affected particularly in cases where the co-twin died (Russell 1961; Griffiths 1967).

Within a pair the smaller of the two at birth is at greater risk (Russell 1961). Again perinatal hazards are in most cases responsible for this high incidence. Griffiths (1967), in her study of 78 twin pairs in which one or both twins had cerebral palsy, found only four instances of concordance but 16 of the children were single surviving twins, their co-twin having been stillborn or having died in the neonatal period. Of those whose twins had died 80% were MZ.

The highest incidence of cerebral palsy was amongst secondborn and breech-delivered infants but she found two distinct neurological pictures amongst the children, depending on their birth order. The firstborn infant who developed cerebral palsy was more likely to have been premature and vertex delivered and characteristically suffered from spastic diplegia. Affected secondborn twins tended to be more mature. In these cases the damage was related to abnormal presentation and birth asphyxia. The result was a more severe form of cerebral palsy such as quadraplegia and/or athetosis.

Similarly Alberman (1964) found a bimodal distribution to cerebral palsy in twins and suggested that there may be two separate aetiological groups. The first group were babies of less than 32 weeks' gestation and the incidence of cerebral palsy in this group was no higher amongst twins than singletons of the same gestational period. However in the second group, whose incidence peaked at 37 weeks' gestational age, the occurrence of cerebral palsy was greatly in excess of that expected in babies of such maturity.

The effects of prematurity, malpresentation and birth asphyxia individually or in combination, have already been discussed. Another aetiological factor peculiar to twinning has been emphasized by Durkin et al. (1976). Of 19 twins with cerebral palsy and severe mental retardation nine had a stillborn co-twin. The author suggests that intrauterine disseminated intravascular coagulation, as a result of a surviving monochorionic fetus sharing a placental circulation with a macerated dead fetus, could have caused the cerebral damage (see p.59).

Most studies on cerebral palsy in twins were reported in the 1960s. With better obstetric and neonatal care both the incidence and pattern are likely now to be changing.

The Handicapped Twin in the Family

The response of a mother to a handicapped child, especially if it is recognizable as such at or soon after birth, may be very similar to that of bereavement. Denial, anger, guilt and grief are all reactions common to both. She mourns for the child that 'might have been'. A mother with one normal twin has no difficulty in imagining what might have been—the image is constantly there. Rather than rejoicing in the normality of the one the mother may, often unconsciously, blame the healthy child for the handicap of the other. Many of her attitudes may be similar to those towards a single surviving twin that will be described in Chapter 13. In the same way the healthy twin may feel both guilt and anger towards his twin. One MZ twin described the sight of his handicapped brother 'like looking in the mirror at a caricature of myself'. There are practical difficulties too. The handicapped twin is likely to take up a disproportionate share of the mother's time and attention. Visits to doctors and therapists may be time-consuming and the problems of taking (or leaving) the healthy twin may, at times, be insurmountable. Every consideration should be given to such families. Arrangements for the care of the healthy twin should be as much the concern of the handicap team as for their patient. It is often quite practical for the twin to join in the activities of some therapy groups. The mother will then be more relaxed and more able to concentrate on the handicapped twin.

Clearly as they grow beyond babyhood the intellectual as well as the physical needs of the two children will increasingly digress. To balance the needs of the handicapped child with those of his sibling is always a problem for parents. With twins there is danger that by emphasizing the twinship the development of the more advanced child may be held back. The needs and particularly the feelings of the healthy twin are often complex and a family may need skilled counselling in coping with them (Bernabei and Levi 1976).

13. Death of a Twin

Many parents of twins have to face the tragedy of bereavement. Not only do they have twice the risk but from the moment of conception, the mortality rate of twins is relatively high.

In early pregnancy an unknown, but large, number of single twins are lost (p.31). Later the risk of intrauterine death is higher than for singletons; higher still is the neonatal mortality rate (p.95). This increased risk of death persists, although at a lower level, at least through the first year of life.

For parents of twins the loss of two babies is a tragedy. For some it is heightened by the shattering of the enormous prestige which society attaches to having twins. But, as the parents gain the admiration, so also will they now gain the sympathy of relatives, of friends and of the medical profession.

Not so the parents who lose one twin; particularly one who was stillborn or died within the first few days. Society, consciously or not, forgets the dead baby. Emotions are concentrated on the surviving child and the parents are encouraged to do the same. The parents are therefore prevented from mourning.

With a single bereavement there is the additional difficulty of having a constant reminder in the survivor of the child that might have been. This is enhanced further in MZ twins. Later the parents will have to cope with the, often complex, feelings of a child deprived of its close partner.

ABORTION AND FETUS PAPYRACEUS

The spontaneous abortion of twins is little, if any, more common than that of singletons. The loss of one of the two fetuses during the first trimester is not, however, unusual (p.31). Before the introduction of ultrasound these twin pregnancies were unrecognized except when a fetus papyraceus was noticed when the single baby was delivered. The only other abnormality might have been a vaginal bleed in the early months.

There are other occasions when a twin pregnancy is missed. Some 'premature' babies, thought to have been conceived immediately after an early abortion, are surprisingly large and mature for their length of gestation. It is likely that at least some of these babies are single survivors of the original (twin) pregnancy.

It is not known how much the early loss of a twin fetus may affect both the mother or indeed the single survivor. There is evidence that at least some twins have personality problems related to the loss of their partner. This may be so even when the survivor is not conscious of having been a twin. It may be more important than now realized that both mother and child should be aware of the twinship (Lewis 1983).

STILLBIRTH AND NEONATAL DEATH

After months of expectation and anticipation of a life-to-be there is no bigger anticlimax than the birth of a dead baby. Society shuns it. Even the medical profession does so. It wraps it up and buries it as soon as possible. It tries its best to forget the baby ever was (Bourne 1968). People manage to do this distressingly soon (for the parents) even with a single baby.

With twins this reality avoidance can be accomplished with even greater ease. Attention to the surviving twin provides an escape route. By concentrating on the live baby it is quite possible, once out of the delivery room, never to mention the lost baby. Some mothers have found that midwives whom they have known well during their pregnancy did not—perhaps could not—even refer to the baby who died.

In fact the mother, and often the father too, wants to talk about the stillborn baby; to ask questions about how and why it happened; to vent anger; to attribute blame; just to share her feelings, rational or not, about the baby she has lost and what he might have been.

Mothers invariably feel shame and to some extent guilt that somehow they are responsible for the baby's death. They may feel they have actually 'killed' their baby. The mother's guilt may be increased by misguided remarks such as, 'How lucky you still have one healthy baby' and 'Two babies would have been such a handful'.

This concentration on the healthy baby to the exclusion of the stillbirth when she is longing to talk about the latter may make the mother idealize the dead one and positively alienate her from the survivor. Its 'normal' crying, feeding habits and restlessness may irritate her quite unreasonably, so much that she may feel it is punishing her. Child abuse would not be unexpected in situations of this kind and has been reported in a surviving twin of a 'cot death' (Bluglass 1980).

It is well known that pregnancy and the arrival of a new baby inhibits mourning (Lewis 1979a). A pregnancy following too soon after a stillbirth may have disastrous consequences. If the mother has not adequately mourned her dead baby she is likely to have serious misidentifications of the new child with its dead sibling (Lewis and Page 1978). Twins are an extreme example of this. The mother experiences the joy of the new life and the tragedy of death simultaneously. She is likely to suppress her grief; those around her encourage her to do so. She may appear to do this successfully for some time but later, sometimes after many years, she may well suffer from severe psychiatric disorders.

Maternity hospital staff should do all they can to facilitate, rather than impede, the normal process of mourning (Lewis 1979b). Suppressing this natural process of grieving and lament is likely to delay acceptance and have damaging results for each parent, for their marriage, and not least for the surviving twin.

It is important that a mother is able clearly to distinguish the two babies in her mind. One mother, who had never seen her stillborn baby, felt that the surviving twin was 'only half a baby' (Lewis 1983). If she had some substantive memories of the dead baby she would have found it easier to avoid the confusion. All parents should be given opportunity, and encouragement, to see the dead baby and indeed to handle it. A photograph should always be taken. Parents who did not see their baby (many are not given the chance to) may treasure this one souvenir. Parents have been known to ask for a photograph years later. When this is not available an x-ray or a photograph of an ultrasound scan can be a great comfort if only to confirm that this nebulous baby did exist. Likewise blood samples should always be taken for zygosity determination. Even if one or both babies die, parents nearly always want to know whether or not their twins were 'identical'. The zygosity may also be essential for reliable genetic counselling particularly if either baby was malformed.

Too often the funeral arrangements are taken over by well-meaning hospital staff and the event minimized in the hope that the whole sad episode will be forgotten. People need to name their child, to have a memorable funeral and an individual grave or memorial.

One mother's feelings about her lost baby were so complex and ran so deep that she found herself unable to arrange the christening for her surviving baby that she would normally have wanted. It was only when it was suggested, 4 years later, that the christening might be combined with a memorial service for the stillborn twin that she felt able to face, indeed welcome, the service.

Similar considerations are relevant when both babies are born alive but one is likely to die soon from, say, gross malformations or severe birth anoxia. In these cases parents are often encouraged to focus their attention on the healthier baby. This they may later regret. A mother wants to do as much for any baby of hers as possible. If his life is to be short there is all the more reason to give him as much love and care while she can, and she then at least has some experiences to remember. Similarly if one twin is on the special care baby unit and the other at her bedside, the mother should always be encouraged to visit and think about the one separated from her. She should never be allowed to feel that her frequent visits or requests for information are in any way a nuisance to the hospital staff.

The need for a mother to talk about her dead baby may be intense during the first weeks. It can be trying for those with her and some may feel critical of her apparent lack of interest in the healthy baby. It may however be necessary for her to come to terms with her dead baby before she can really bond to the survivor, and her needs should be respected. It is only by allowing, indeed encouraging, her to think and talk about the baby that the normal mourning process can take place.

Most mothers continue to welcome opportunities to reminisce about the baby who died, particularly with those who were with her at the time of her bereavement, sometimes for many years. Paediatricians, family doctors and clinical medical officers should make clear to the mother that she is welcome to do so. It is good practice for the paediatrician to see the mother and, if possible the father too, with the surviving twin on at least one occasion in his follow-up clinic, even if it is not medically necessary. He will then be able to make sure that she is happy with the baby's progress and it will also give her the chance to ask any questions about the dead twin—or just to talk about him and about her feelings of loss.

SUDDEN INFANT DEATH SYNDROME

The sudden unexpected death of a baby is a shattering experience for any parent. Four in every thousand families suffer the tragedy of Sudden Infant Death Syndrome (SIDS), otherwise known as a 'cot death', in the UK. The incidence amongst twins is higher still partly, but probably not entirely, due to the adverse factors known to be associated with both twinning and SIDS such as prematurity and low birth weight (see p.119).

Parents usually feel extreme guilt, however unjustified. They may believe that something they did or failed to do must have been responsible for the death. This belief is often reinforced by the bewildered and embarrassed attitudes of their relatives and neighbours which the parents interpret as criticism of their care and confirmation of their guilt. The mother is determined that the same should not happen to the other baby.

Many parents are so obsessed by the fear of the survivor's demise that they are unable to let him out of their sight. The slightest abnormal sign or symptom results in urgent calls to the doctor or hospital. The parents become so exhausted by the strain and lack of sleep that the baby's admission to hospital for a few days, together with his mother, may be the only way to ease the tension and allow the mother some much needed sleep. This may also give her the opportunity to talk over the many worries and unanswered questions that always accompany a SIDS.

The whole family will need support and understanding often lasting for many months and years. Easy access to and frequent visits from the health visitor are often welcomed. The health visitor will, of course, need sensitivity and tact to ensure that her attentions are seen as being supportive rather than an indication of the mother's failure to care for her child on her own.

Many surviving babies appear deeply affected by the death of their twin even when they are only a few months old. In part this must be due to the general family upset and the change in mood and attitude of their parents. Nevertheless the event itself may be of deeper significance to the co-twin than, at present, realized. One mother described the shocked expression and ashen complexion of the healthy twin as she lay in the same cot beside her dead sister. It was the appearance of the first baby that led the mother to look at the dead one.

When so little is known about the causes of SIDS parents find comfort in the knowledge that many other apparently healthy babies with caring parents die in the same way. They often appreciate introductions to other bereaved parents either locally or through the Association for the Study of SIDS (see address list).

DEATH IN CHILDHOOD

Twins are little if any more likely to die in childhood than singletons. But for those who do—be it from accidents, chronic illness or acute infections—the effects on the survivor can be devastating (Bernabei and Levi 1976). This is particularly so if the twins had had little experience of being separated or if the one who died was the 'leader'. For these children the beliefs of some African tribes that the spirit of the dead twin must be preserved in order to ensure the wholeness of the survivor may appear frighteningly apt (Chapter 1).

Many survivors feel a guilt that they were the one chosen to live. This guilt, of course, is compounded if they think that they were directly—or even indirectly—responsible for their twin's death.

Young children have great difficulty in understanding the finality of death, that their brother or sister will never return. One 3-year-old, whose brother had died in hospital 6 months earlier, insisted on taking some of his toys to the doctor at Christmas-time so that they could be given to his twin. For all ages it is nearly always helpful for them to be as much involved in the terminal illness and death of their sibling, as well as mourning, as reasonably possible. The unknown and unseen is more frightening and incomprehensible than reality. For a twin this must be particularly important. With the chronically ill child there are advantages both to him and his healthy twin of being together through the final weeks. Janet Goodall and the parents concerned have sensitively and revealingly described how a family coped with the terminal illness of a 5-year-old at home rather than in hospital. This clearly enabled the older and younger sisters to accept and come to terms with the death of their brother more easily than they would otherwise have done had they been excluded from the whole experience (Cotton et al. 1981).

Many parents, whilst still grieving themselves, find the disturbances in behaviour of the surviving twin particularly distressing. One 2½-year-old suddenly lost his MZ twin brother from bacterial meningitis. Having had normal speech development as well as an elaborate 'twin language' he became silent. Six weeks later his mother took him to the mirror to point out some dirty marks on his face. His expression lit up for a few seconds only to turn to anguish as he realized the reflection was his own, not his twin. He refused to go near a mirror again and became increasingly withdrawn and destructive. Other times there may be profound psychic injuries that do not show any immediate overt symptoms.

Some children's behaviour at these times can be so difficult as to seriously disrupt family life. Parents, although both anxious to help their unhappy child, may disagree profoundly on the best method of so doing. Marital discord is common. It is vital that all families should be offered support and bereavement counselling from the earliest possible moment in the hope of preventing or at least reducing both the child's difficulties and the family tensions.

MOTHER'S ATTITUDE TO THE SURVIVING TWIN

Most mothers have ambivalent feelings towards the surviving twin. Some overprotect the survivor. Others reject. Many do both. They are thankful to have this baby (or child) to love and yet they often feel that he is in some way responsible for the death of the other. Perhaps he had an unfair share of intrauterine nutrition. With an older child the mother may feel that an accident which killed one was the fault of the other. Sometimes, of course, this is true.

Many parents are haunted by the vision of their dead child in the living twin. One mother dreaded washing her 2-year-old's hair for it was when his hair was wet that he looked most like his dead brother. Another mother described how her 18-month-old daughter acquired a number of mannerisms peculiar to her dead MZ twin which she herself had never before shown. These ever-present reminders of the lost child can be so painful that the mother, at least temporarily, rejects the twin and may give an unfair amount of attention to the siblings. Even with a stillborn baby this same problem may arise. One mother who had never seen the stillborn baby found that each time she looked at his live twin she was unable to stop herself wondering what the dead one was like.

In their dreams of the child that should have been many mothers idealize the dead baby and as the survivor fails to live up to the image of his twin the mother may become excessively critical of his 'faults'. Scapegoating of a surviving twin to the extent of physical and mental abuse has been described by Bluglass (1980).

A mother's guilt in failing to produce a live baby may be

increased further by her apparent inability to care for the survivor. Through the projection of her own anxieties the baby becomes increasingly 'difficult'. Her humiliation is complete when the baby calms on being handled by the father or other caretakers. She becomes severely depressed and may abandon the baby altogether (Lewis and Page 1978).

Expert and prolonged psychiatric help is often needed for the whole family.

The Father

In general it is believed that mothers feel the loss of a baby or young child more deeply than the father. The reverse, however, may be true with an older child (Bowlby 1980). But whatever his feelings about the actual bereavement the father will need a lot of support in coping with the mother's grief and the reactions of the surviving twin. He often finds it harder to express his own grief and society reinforces these inhibitions by concentrating its sympathy on the mother.

Most fathers are extremely proud of having twins and in the early months many think of them as a single unit. The destruction of this unit leaves an incomplete child, one whom the father may now reject. After the loss of a 2-year-old twin son the father insisted on the removal of all photographs of the pair. He was able to give his love and attention to the 5-year-old sister but wanted nothing to do with the MZ twin who was too painful a reminder of the lost son.

THE SURVIVING TWIN

The sense of loss and incompleteness felt by a surviving twin who has lost his twin at birth are illuminated in the Italian novel *I fantasmi della mia vita* by Achille Geremicca. As a child the subject had longed for a companion to strengthen and comfort him; he had even created an imaginary twin. Later he discovered that he was in fact a single surviving twin—'a poor survivor, a remaining soul, a mutilated life, a mere half which, by itself, is as sad as a ruin'.

The number of single surviving twins in the UK is difficult to determine. National perinatal mortality figures distinguish between singletons and twins but they do not reveal the number of twin pairs in which only one twin died.

On the assumption that twins who have been brought up on their own have lost their co-twin through death then a figure of 15% for single survivors can be deduced from the study by Record et al. (1970) on 2164 twins taking the eleven-plus examination. A more recent study found that 10% of 5½- to 7½-year-old twin pairs had only one surviving child (Phillips and Watkinson 1981). The lower rates of 5–9% have been found in several studies of single twin survivors up to the end of the perinatal period, by which time the great majority of deaths would have occurred (Potter 1963; Ferguson 1964; Hendricks 1966; Myrianthopoulos 1970).

The price of being a single survivor may be very high. Some of the problems of the surviving twin both in his relationship with his parents and with himself have already been discussed. Many are still ill understood.

There seems no doubt, however, that overt psychiatric morbidity is higher in single surviving twins than in either the general population or in twins whose co-twin is still alive. Twenty-six per cent of twin-born patients attending the Maudsley Psychiatric Hospital in London had lost their co-twin and amongst those with psychotic illness the figure rose to 44% (Reveley et al. 1981).

To be the twin of a stillborn baby may be the worst catastrophe of all. Many survivors appear to carry the onus for their twin's death right into adulthood. This guilt may be expressed in their relationships with others. They tend to compensate by looking after and marrying people weaker than themselves. They may have a morbid preoccupation with death. One survivor arranged a suicide pact with his brother, thereby repeating history.

Even those twins who appear psychologically and socially unscathed may suffer profoundly from their bereavement.

A 58-year-old head school teacher had lost her MZ twin at the age of 6 weeks. Despite a large family she greatly missed her twin and now describes her 'desperate sense of loss and loneliness' throughout childhood which she revealed to no one. She also had fantasies that the dead twin was still alive; these continued until adolescence. Even as an adult she continued to dream of her lost twin.

Too often the dead twin is never mentioned. It is rare, for instance, for a teacher at school, or even in a playgroup, to know of a twin who died at birth or soon after. Yet the child's first drawings may show that he needs to express his twinship. Perhaps there is the recurring second figure. Other times the loss may be demonstrated by incomplete bodies or even objects with missing parts.

One 3-year-old, whose twin was stillborn, was repeatedly attracted to depleted objects (Lewis 1983)—the toy car without a wheel, the doll with a missing arm.

All single surviving twins should hear about their dead twins from the start and be encouraged to ask questions and express their feelings, rational or not. Many feel angry: angry with the twin for deserting them, for causing such unhappiness in the family, for making them, the survivors, feel guilty. They may also feel anger towards their parents for 'allowing' the twin to die. Some have secret fantasies which can be frightening and indeed dangerous if allowed to develop.

SUPPORT FROM SELF-HELP GROUPS

Most parents continue to think of their single surviving child as a twin even if the co-twin was stillborn, and they like other people to do the same. For this reason some parents continue to join in the activities of their local twins club. Others, not surprisingly, find the contact with twins and their parents too painful but welcome a chance to share their feelings with other bereaved parents, particularly those who had twins.

The national Twins Clubs Association provides introductions to parents in similar situations. Likewise the Stillborn and Perinatal Death Association and the Foundation for the Study of Infant Deaths gives useful information, guidance and contact with other bereaved families. Other organizations such as the Compassionate Friends can be a great comfort to some families. Addresses of these organizations are given in the Appendix.

14. Higher Multiple Births

Although this book is about twins it would be incomplete without some consideration of higher multiple births. Families with 'supertwins' have most of the same experiences and share most of the same problems—some of them, of course, with greater intensity.

There is theoretically no limit to the number of infants that a human mother can produce at one delivery. Hoaxers, mythologists and imaginative historians have made the most of this fact. Mayer (1952a,b) comprehensively reviewed all reports of sextuplets or more, whether they were authentic or legendary, and found at least eight examples of the delivery of ten or more infants. One claim was of 365! Traditionally the delivery of multiple offspring has been regarded as a punishment for a number of misdemeanors, sexual or other.

Rare but authentic cases of multiple births as high as seven have been reported in the past (Mayer 1952b). The incidence of these very high multiples has however greatly increased since the introduction of ovulation-stimulating drugs for the treatment of infertility.

A case of nonoplets, none of whom survived, is probably the largest recorded multiple birth (Benirschke and Kim 1973). Octuplets, of whom seven are said to have survived, were reported to have been born 120 miles from Shanghai. However, the report comes indirectly from the father via an Italian newspaper and has not been confirmed (Mayer 1952b). An octuplet abortion has been reliably reported (Prokop and Herrmann 1973). There have been a number of septuplet pregnancies. Most ended in abortion or neonatal death (Mayer 1952*b*; Turksoy et al. 1967; Burnell 1974); in a few cases some of the infants have survived (Aiken 1969).

Giovannucci-Uzielli et al. (1981) claim that the 'Florentine' sextuplets (Fig. 14.1) are the first to survive the neonatal period. Certainly they appear to be the first corroborated in the medical press. However, it seems that all the Bushnell sextuplets, born in Chicago in 1866, were alive at 8 months. Amazingly they escaped

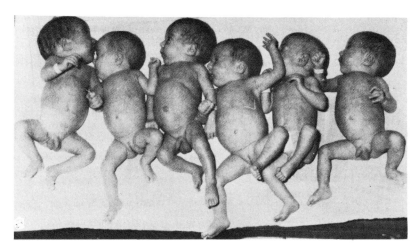

Fig. 14.1. The 'Florentine' sextuplets born at 34 weeks' gestation. Four boys weighing 1430 g, 1520 g, 1540 g, 1700 g and two girls each weighing 1150 g. There were six chorionic membranes in the single placental mass. From Giovannucci-Uzielli et al. (1981) by permission of Alan R. Liss.

publicity and the three survivors were only 'discovered' at the age of 72. Apparently one girl and one boy had died at 8 months and a second brother at the age of 68 years (Mayer 1952*a*). Lachelin et al. (1972) reported sextuplets of whom five survived.

A number of surviving quintuplets have now been reported (McArthur 1937; Liggins and Ibbertson 1966; Campbell and Dewhurst 1970; Jewelewicz et al. 1972). Many of their mothers were on treatment for infertility but several have been spontaneous pregnancies. The most famous are of course the Dionne quintuplets who were exceptional in being monozygotic (McArthur 1937). The surviving set reported by Campbell and Dewhurst (1970) had the advantage of close supervision throughout their intrauterine life as they were diagnosed by ultrasound as early as 9 weeks.

INCIDENCE

Pregnancies with more than three fetuses are so rare as to make incidences calculated on such small numbers meaningless. In England and Wales in 1979 figures for multiple births where there was at least one liveborn infant included six sets of quadruplets, 76 of triplets and 6099 pairs of twins (Registrar General 1979). A set of quintuplets was born in 1978 and sextuplets in 1976. Hellin (1895) proposed a formula by which the frequency of higher multiple births in a given population could be calculated and this has since become known as Hellin's law. If n is the frequency of twins in a population, n^2 is that of triplets, n^3 of quadruplets and so on. Hellin did not take into account the zygosity distributions in different populations. [Several workers have suggested modifications to the calculation to allow for this (Nylander 1975b)]. Nevertheless Hellin's law remains useful in indicating the probable range of higher multiple births within a given population.

In countries like the UK where the incidence of twins is approximately 1 in 100 deliveries then that of triplets should be 1 in 10 000 and that of quadruplets 1 in 1 000 000. Thus according to Hellin's law no more than one set of quadruplets would be expected each year in the UK, whereas in practice there was an average of over five sets a year between 1971 and 1979. Treatment for infertility is probably responsible for this high incidence.

In a study of 2369 pregnancies resulting from treatment with Clomid (clomiphene citrate) the incidence of twins was 6.9%, triplets 0.5%, quadruplets 0.3% and quintuplets 0.13% (Merrell Pharmaceuticals Ltd. 1981).

Factors influencing the incidence of higher multiple births are the same as those for twins and are outlined in Chapter 2. There are many reports of triplets occurring in the same family as twins (Miettinen 1954). As would be expected the incidence of triplets amongst negro races is much higher than amongst Caucasians and an incidence of two per 1000 has been reported from Nigeria (Nylander 1971a). Even so this is not nearly as high as the six per 1000 predicted by Hellin's law. A high undetected abortion rate could explain the discrepancy, at least in part.

TYPES OF HIGHER MULTIPLE BIRTHS

'Supertwins', the term used by Scheinfeld (1973) to describe higher multiple births, may be derived from separate zygotes, or from a

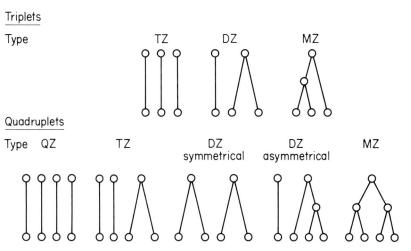

Fig. 14.2. Types of triplets and quadruplets.

single zygote or from a combination of the two. The possible combinations in a triplet and quadruplet set are shown in Fig. 14.2. DZ triplets, for example, are derived from two zygotes, one of which later divides into an MZ pair.

Combinations for the higher multiples can be worked out from the basic triplet and quadruplet patterns.

Zygosity

In many higher multiple births the zygosity of the babies has not been accurately determined. There are therefore few data on the relative frequency of the different types. It has been estimated that the ratio of MZ: DZ: TZ triplets amongst Caucasians should be 1 : 2 : 3 and details of the calculations are given by Bulmer (1970). Some studies however have found higher incidences of DZ triplets than would be expected (Bulmer 1970).

Amongst mongolian races, such as the Japanese, the proportion of MZ triplets is of course much higher whereas TZ triplets are proportionately more common amongst negro races. Of 40 sets of triplets born in Ibaden, Western Nigeria, only two were MZ and 24 were TZ (Nylander and Corney 1971).

MZ quadruplets and quintuplets are rare but have been authentically reported (McArthur 1938; B. Martin 1981, personal communication) (Fig. 14.3). DZ quadruplets may be asymmetrical with three infants arising from one zygote or symmetrical when two

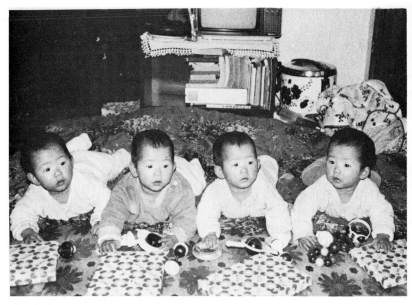

Fig. 14.3. MZ quadruplets from South Korea. By permission of Dr. B. Martin.

zygotes split to form MZ pairs. Only occasional examples of the latter have been reported (Nylander and Corney 1971).

Most ovulation-induced pregnancies resulting in higher multiple births are polyzygotic but, interestingly, the numbers which also include an MZ pair appear to be higher than would be expected by chance (Atlay and Pennington 1971). It has been suggested that polyovulation may in itself promote division of the zygote (Benirschke and Kim 1973).

Sex

MZ triplets must be the same sex whereas half DZ sets will be of like sex and only one quarter of TZ.

The sex ratio in triplets is even lower than that found in twins (see p.11). This higher proportion of females may be due to an increase in abortions of the more vulnerable male (Bulmer 1970).

PREGNANCY

The reaction of parents when told that they are to have more than two babies is even more ambivalent than that of parents of twins.

They are excited by the novelty and prestige even if they are apprehensive about publicity. Most of them are worried by the practical and financial implications. Those that are not are either unrealistic or blessed with exceptional financial and practical support.

The chance of losing some, if not all, the babies is high and most parents realize this. Many couples will have had several years of infertility and thus the prospect of a ready made family is particularly attractive. On the other hand their fear for the babies' safety is bound to be all the greater because of the difficulty they have had in conceiving.

A triplet pregnancy is uncomfortable at the very least. Complications are common and all those discussed in Chapter 3 are even more likely to occur in higher multiple than in twin pregnancies. Most mothers will need periods of bedrest, usually in hospital. All should be delivered in centres with facilities for intensive care of the infants.

Fetal hazards peculiar to multiple pregnancies such as the fetofetal transfusion syndromes (Cortes 1964), monoamniotic placentation (Sinykin 1958; Wharton et al. 1968) and locking have all been reported amongst higher multiple births as well as the congenital malformations discussed below.

Duration of Pregnancy

Any factors which predispose to preterm delivery of twins have even greater effect in a higher multiple pregnancy. Despite the slower fetal growth during the third trimester, the total fetal and placental weight in triplets or more will be considerably greater— as will the uterine distension—than in twins.

The average duration of pregnancy in triplets is about 247 days and of quadruplets 237 (McKeown and Record 1952) compared with 260 days in twins and 280 in singletons.

Delivery

Most obstetricians are happy to deliver triplets vaginally as long as there are no complications. For quadruplets or more many prefer to perform an elective caesarean section (MacGillivray 1975*b*). The famous Dionne quintuplets were remarkable in all being delivered spontaneously at home, with no apparent complications (McArthur 1937).

As birth asphyxia and extreme prematurity are common, at least one paediatrician with full equipment for resuscitation should be available for each baby.

Birth Weight

McKeown and Record (1952) were the first to point out that the greater the number of babies, the lower were their individual birth weights (Fig. 14.4). They found that the average birth weight for

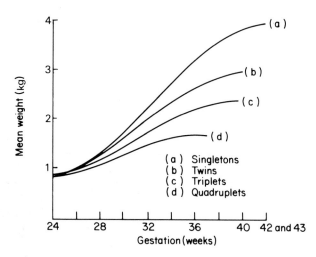

Fig. 14.4. Birth weights of multiple births in relation to gestation. From MacGillivray (1975*c*) by permission of the author and W.B. Saunders Co. Ltd.

triplets was 1.8 kg, and for quadruplets 1.4 kg. Others have reported similar results for triplets (Bulmer 1970). Whatever the number of fetuses it seems that all grow at a similar rate to singletons until the latter part of the second trimester. Only then does growth slow down in direct relation to the number of fetuses that the uteroplacental circulation must supply.

Congenital Malformations

There have been many instances in which one or more members of a higher multiple set is malformed. Burnell (1974) reported two anencephalics in a set of otherwise normal septuplets; all three fetuses were affected in MZ triplets (Scott and Paterson 1966). A conjoined pair may have a normal third partner (Tan et al. 1971;

Vestergaard 1972). An acardiac monster may be part of a monochorionic pair with a third dichorionic unaffected fetus (Benirschke and Kim 1973).

PLACENTATION

Accurate descriptions of placentae in higher multiple births tend to be limited to case reports. There have been detailed descriptions of several types including the placenta of septuplets (Cameron et al. 1969; Fig. 14.5). Little attention, however, has been given to the

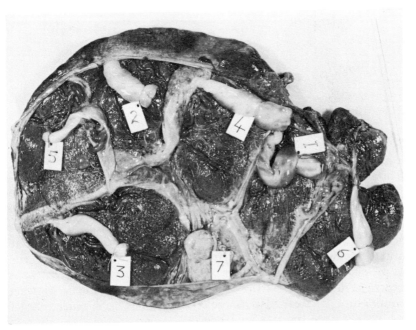

Fig. 14.5. Placenta from a septuplet pregnancy. None of the six liveborn infants were monozygotic and seven chorionic sacs were present. There were three females and four males, one of whom was a fetus papyraceus. From Cameron et al. (1969) by permission of the authors and the editors of *Journal of Obstetrics and Gynaecology of the British Commonwealth.*

frequency of the various chorion types as in most studies the numbers, even of triplets, are too small.

Following the pattern described for twins in Chapter 6 the placentae of all TZ triplets will be dichorionic, one-third of DZ triplets should also have three chorions whereas two-thirds will be dichorionic. On the same grounds one-ninth of MZ triplets should

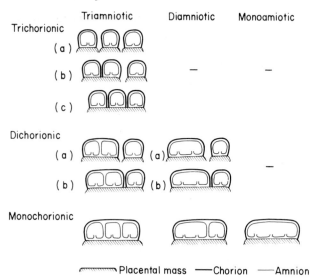

Fig. 14.6. The different types of triplet placentae. From Nylander and Corney (1971) by permission of the authors and the editors of *Annals of Human Genetics*.

be trichorionic, four-ninths dichorionic and four-ninths monochorionic. These various types of placentation are shown in Fig. 14.6. Those for higher multiple births can be deduced from this.

The actual number of each chorion type will of course depend on the proportion of TZ triplets in the population. In a total of 23 sets of Caucasian triplets collected from the literature there were equal numbers (eight) of trichorionic and dichorionic placentae and three monochorionic (Nylander and Corney 1971). In Nigeria, as would be expected, the percentage of trichorionic placentae is much higher than in the UK. In 40 sets of triplets 29 were trichorionic, 10 were dichorionic and only one was monochorionic.

NEWBORN 'SUPERTWINS'

For all parents of 'supertwins' the first weeks are a strain. The mother is recovering from what is likely to have been a tiring pregnancy and a difficult delivery. There is nearly always medical concern about at least one of the babies and sometimes about all of them. The mother may well try to prevent herself becoming attached to these babies to save herself from grief should they die. She often has to lament the loss of one baby either as a stillbirth or as a neonatal death, while she is still anxious for the life of the others. The uncertainty of the first days or weeks as one baby after another dies can be an intolerable strain. For those parents who are left with one or more survivors there is a complex process of celebrating the lives of some and grieving the death of others (see Chapter 13). For those who have two or more survivors society (indeed logic) suggests that the family has had enough additions as it is. Nevertheless the mother has lost a precious baby and her grief should not be denied or minimized. Few counsellors will have had experience with this unusual situation and often the best support for this kind of bereaved family comes from other parents who have experienced it.

Perinatal Mortality

The perinatal mortality rate amongst higher multiple births is, of course, very high. So far there have probably been only two sets of sextuplets to survive the neonatal period (Mayer 1952*a*; Giovannucci-Uzielli et al. 1981). Whole quintuplet sets are rare and even sets of quadruplets are usually incomplete. Perinatal mortality rates in these higher multiple births are bound to be inaccurate owing to the small numbers, but the stillbirth rate in quadruplets has been estimated as about six times that of singletons (Miettinen 1954; Heady and Heasman 1955) and their neonatal mortality rate is much higher still. Patten (1970) found that triplets had a perinatal mortality rate of 118 per 1000 compared with 48 per 1000 in singletons. Others have found the relative difference to be even greater (Miettinen 1954; Heady and Heasman 1955). The main cause of death is, as in twins, that of prematurity. But the other complications described in Chapters 4 and 5 apply at least as often to all the higher multiple births.

Most, if not all, parents will be aware of the high risk associated with a multiple pregnancy. For many this will be a constant if often unspoken anxiety throughout their pregnancy—a pregnancy which is already likely to be distressing due to complications or, at the very least, great discomfort. Some have to face the loss of all babies, a particularly cruel blow to those couples who had waited long for this pregnancy (Burnell 1974).

MANAGEMENT

Some mothers cope adequately, even well, with twins on their own. But with triplets help is essential at least during the first year. Even if a mother can manage the numerous practical needs of three babies, her inability to respond simultaneously to their demands makes the emotional burden impossible for one to carry alone. Two babies can, for example, be comforted at the same time. There is no arm left for a third.

Thus arrangements for regular help are a first priority with triplets. Labour-saving devices should be welcomed and any 'time savers' suggested for twins (see p.113) become even more valuable.

Feeding

There is no way a mother can feed more than two babies at the same time (except by propping the bottles, a practice which is to be strongly discouraged). Help with at least some feeds is essential if she is not to spend most of her day on feeding rounds. Many mothers have partially breast-fed their triplets. Very occasionally they have been entirely breast-fed (Noble 1980). Some mothers will breast-feed two at each feed whilst a helper gives a bottle to the third baby.

One mother of 'quads' chose to breast-feed one baby only at each feed. This meant that all four babies had their mother's undivided attention for at least half an hour each day. She felt that this was the only way she could develop a strong relationship with each baby. She was of course fortunate in having a willing team to feed the other three.

Transport

Transport of the babies is always a problem. Initially a large twin pram will suffice with two babies at one end. Some mothers prefer to carry one of the babies in a sling at both the pram and early pushchair stages. Apart from the convenience, this allows the mother a little extra time of physical contact which is always in short supply. A triplet buggy can be formed by clipping a single onto a twin buggy (Fig. 14.7). The Twins Clubs Association has an especially adapted foursome pram which can be hired for quadruplets.

It is difficult, indeed sometimes impossible, to keep an eye on three active babies. For this reason many mothers restrict triplets more than they would a single child. Goshen-Gottstein (1980) found that triplets were confined to playpens or even cots for long periods of the day. Many children missed out on the early

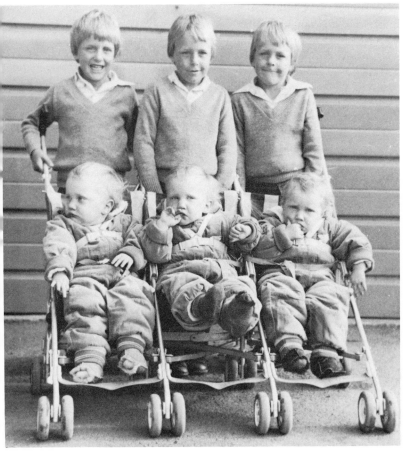

Fig. 14.7. Two sets of triplets—the older boys are dizygotic and the younger girls are monozygotic.

exploration which is an important part of any child's development (Fig. 14.8).

MOTHERS' ATTITUDES

Even if their initial reaction to the idea of twins was negative most mothers happily accept their two babies by the time they are born—or at least soon afterwards. But Goshen-Gottstein (1980) found that this was not necessarily so with mothers of supertwins. Seven out of ten mothers of triplets and quadruplets remained

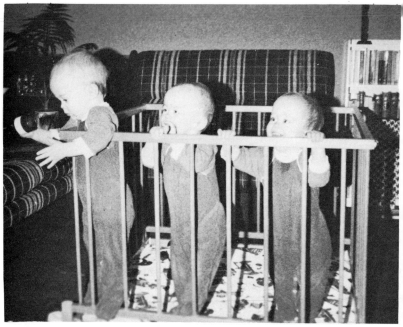

Fig. 14.8. Triplets in playpen.

upset throughout the early months. However, several of these Israeli mothers already had large families when the supertwins arrived. In the UK, where families tend to be smaller, it may well be that more mothers would have a positive approach.

The greater the number of babies the harder it is for a mother to relate to each individually. Responding to the particular needs of each baby at the same time is an enormous strain. Many parents resort to treating them all alike with no regard for their different personalities. They tend to assume that their needs must be the same. That all should eat the same amount, that if one is tired then they must all be. They may make little effort to distinguish the babies either by name or dress. To dress all babies differently demands imagination and energy.

There seems to be advantages in being the 'odd-one-out' either in sex or zygosity. That child has more chance of being treated as an individual. Many mothers treat like-sexed and in particular MZ children as a unit and refer to them as such whereas the opposite-sexed child is named. Some mothers with like-sexed DZ triplets dressed only the MZ pair alike thereby actually accentuating the similarity (Goshen-Gottstein 1980).

When several children are competing for their mother's attention the loudest and most persistent tends to win. The noise particularly during the second and third years may be deafening. Many mothers find this in itself a great strain. The price of peace is often the loss of normal discipline and reasoning. Parents tend to swing from appeasement to reprimand without explanation.

Even the most competent mother may find she reaches the end of her tether when one or more are ill. The extra demands of miserable children plus the knowledge that they need and deserve extra love and attention tries the most patient mother.

LONG-TERM DEVELOPMENT

There is no doubt that many members of triplet, quadruplet and even quintuplet sets become healthy adults of normal intelligence. However there have been no large studies that compared the overall development of 'supertwins' with those of singletons. In those that have the numbers are inevitably small.

Miettinen and Grönroos (1965) studied the 225 members of 75 complete sets of triplets, many of whom had been born long before neonatal intensive care was available. Their ages ranged from 3 to 45 years. Nevertheless they found that all but eight (4%) were of normal intelligence. Of the eight, five had a moderate degree of intellectual impairment and three were severely mentally retarded.

The growth of the group as a whole was similar to that of the singleton population. A further finding was that of a twofold increase in lefthandedness in triplets when compared with singletons.

The large Birmingham study of children taking the eleven-plus examination in the 1950s included 33 triplets. The mean IQ of these children was 91.6 compared with 95.7 in twins and 100.1 in singletons.

No detailed study of language development in triplets has been reported. It would not be surprising if language delay in triplets was even greater than that found in twins. Not only do triplets communicate less with their mother but they are also deprived of the one-to-one relationship found in a pair of twins. It would be interesting to know the relative progress of single surviving triplets, members of a pair of surviving triplets and members of a complete set. The handicap of being brought up a twin is likely to be magnified for a triplet, who has two other companions competing for attention.

15. Twins Worldwide

The worldwide interest in twins has been discussed in Chapter 1. Although there may be some remote areas where multiple births are still feared twins are now generally accepted and even welcomed.

In many areas the feelings towards twins have changed even in this generation. In South Korea for instance multiple births used to be a cause for shame and the babies were often rejected. Now they

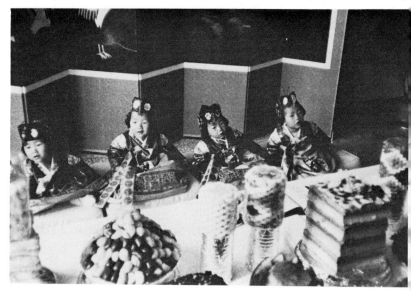

Fig. 15.1. MZ South Korean quadruplets on their first birthday, dressed in national costume. By permission of Dr. B. Martin.

180

are welcomed, at least in the more urbanized, or more westernized communities (Fig. 15.1).

Whatever the attitudes towards twins as a phenomenon, as individual babies they continue to demand special attention. In developed countries they remain an obstetric and paediatric challenge. They are still greatly over-represented in the perinatal mortality and morbidity leagues. On the positive side they are a gift to geneticists and to all who seek enlightenment on the relative effects of heredity and environment. In Third World countries, in addition to the perinatal problems, twins may be a severe drain on a poor family's resources. In areas where the mother is needed to do heavy manual labour, fetching water or gathering wood, often with a baby on her back, she may be unable to continue if she has twins.

In many of these, usually large, families each successive child has its role in relation to the rest. Twins may upset the balance. However West African families in particular are used to the problem; it is not uncommon for a Nigerian mother, for example, to have two or more sets of twins.

Many developing countries cope with twins far better than we do. The extended family is still strong. A grandmother or aunt is usually available to help with the babies. In South Korea, where nearly all babies are transported on a mother's back, I never once saw a mother carrying two babies. A grandmother, aunt or, very often, an older sister was always available to carry the second baby. Breast milk is the only safe nourishment for many Third World babies. A malnourished mother's supply may be inadequate to sustain two babies. However there is often a lactating member of the family or of the village who is willing to provide the necessary supplement.

As extended families dwindle the need for help and support increases. One reflection of this is the emergence of many self-help organizations, not least those for parents of twins. The US led the way and has for many years had Mothers of Twins clubs throughout the country. Other countries are rapidly following suit.

NATIONAL ORGANIZATIONS FOR TWINS AND THEIR FAMILIES

UK—The Twins Clubs Association (TCA) (Fig. 15.2)

The Twins Clubs Association was founded in 1978 by June Tatch with the aim of giving practical and emotional support to families

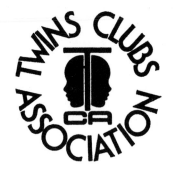

Fig. 15.2. Logo of the Twins Clubs Association

with twins (or more) and to promote understanding of their problems. At the time there were just 12 independent local clubs in the UK, the first of which was established about 10 years earlier By 1982 there were over 150 clubs. The full aims of the TCA are shown in Table 15.1.

Within the Association there is a medical and educational group consisting of parents who are members of medical, paramedical or teaching professions. Members meet regularly to educate themselves and thereafter give lectures to both professional and lay audiences. The group has produced a number of leaflets on the care of twins as well as the *Guide for Mothers of Twins* (Linney 1980b).

Table 15.1. Aims of the Twins Clubs Association

1. To give encouragement and support to parents of twins, triplets and more
2. To publish a National Register of Twins Clubs
3. To promote and establish future clubs
4. To produce and disseminate helpful information and literature to members
5. To increase public and commercial awareness of the special needs of twins and their families
6. To promote greater appreciation within the medical profession of the problems of multiple births
7. To raise funds to promote the above aims

Within the TCA there are subgroups for families of twins in special situations who are less likely to find similar families in a local club. One is concerned with handicapped twins. It keeps a confidential register of those parents who would like to meet families with a similarly handicapped twin(s).

Another group is for parents of adopted twins. This can be particularly helpful in advising prospective adopters as well as social workers on what is involved in the care of twin children. A third group is for single parent families. Another which is of particular value is that for parents who have lost a twin. It is often difficult for a local club to help but through the TCA bereaved families can be put in touch with each other.

A large and active group, founded by Kathy Topping, is one for higher multiple births—the supertwins group. Members can share experiences, exchange equipment and obtain information from a recently produced booklet on the care of supertwins (Topping 1982).

Members of the TCA have cooperated in a number of scientific twin studies and research workers regularly discuss their work at the twice-yearly national conferences. A twice-yearly newsletter is circulated to all members.

USA—National Organization of Mothers of Twins Clubs (NOMOTC)

This, the first national organization for mothers of twins, was founded in 1960 and is now supported by over 200 local clubs with a total membership of nearly 8000.

NOMOTC cooperates in a large number of research and educational projects and publishes *Research in Review* in addition to the quarterly newsletter *MOTC's Notebook*. A 4-day convention is held annually.

A 'Cope/Outreach' committee has recently been formed to help families with special problems.

Canada—Parents of Multiple Births Association (POMBA)

POMBA was founded in 1977 and now has a membership of over 40 clubs and 3000 individuals. It publishes a quarterly newsletter *Double Feature* as well as a variety of leaflets (some also in French).

POMBA gives a special service to higher multiple births. The first publication specifically for quadruplets—the result of an international collaborative study—is in preparation. A 3-day convention is held each May.

Japan—Mothers of Twins Club

Despite the relatively low incidence of multiple births Japan was

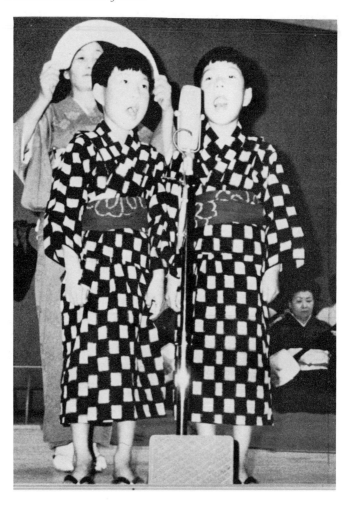

Fig. 15.3. Japanese twins at a Twins Club celebration. By permission of Mrs Y. Amon.

one of the first countries to start self-help clubs for mothers of twins. The national organization was founded in 1968 and there are now over one thousand members (see Fig. 15.3). Each of their two monthly newsletters focusses on a particular aspect of twinning and a compendium of these topics is in preparation. The organization has been involved with a number of research projects and educational meetings are held regularly.

South Africa—South African Multiple Births Association (SAMBA).

This association is largely run on a regional basis with the national organization acting as a coordinating and policy making body. It also produced a twice yearly newsletter, *Gemini Review*.

The association was started in 1976 and now has local clubs in most of the larger towns.

Other Associations

A number of other countries have started self-help organizations for parents of twins. These include Australia (Australian Multiple Birth Association—AMBA), New Zealand (The New Zealand Multiple Births Association), France and Holland (Nederlandse Vereniging van Tweelingen). The addresses of all these are given in the Appendix.

TWIN RESEARCH

Whatever the feelings about twins their special presence cannot be ignored. This book does not propose to discuss the full range of twin studies which have been and still are being carried out. Interest in these has continued and expanded since the pioneering work of Francis Galton (see Chapter 1). Mention must just be made of the International Society for Twin Studies which has done so much to promote the science of twins.

The International Society for Twin Studies (ISTS)

The ISTS is a multidisciplinary scientific organization whose objectives are to 'further research and social action in all fields related to twins and twin studies, for the mutual benefit of the twins and their families and of scientific research' (Constitution of the ISTS 1975).

It was founded in 1974 at the first international congress on twin studies in Rome. Twins, their parents and anyone concerned with twin research are eligible for membership. Scientific members include Geneticists, Psychologists, Psychiatrists, Obstetricians and Paediatricians.

The society publishes a journal *Acta Geneticae Medicae and Gemellologiae* and an international congress is held every third year. The fourth will be in London in 1983.

Appendix

USEFUL ADDRESSES

Twins Clubs Association	2 Steele Rd, London W4, England
International Society for Twin Studies	Piazza Galeno, 5-00161 Rome, Italy
International Society for Twin Studies (Collective Members)	283 7th Avenue S, Lethbridge, Alberta, Canada
Australian Multiple Birth Association	P.O. Box 151, Panania 2213, NSW, Australia
Parents of Multiple Births Association of Canada	283 7th Avenue S, Lethbridge, Alberta, Canada
Mothers of Twins Association of South Africa	112 4th Avenue, Fairland 2195, Johannesburg, Republic of South Africa
National Organization of Mothers of Twins Clubs	5402 Amberwood Lane, Rockville, USA
The New Zealand Multiple Births Association	26 Nelson Street, Greymouth, New Zealand

Nederlandse Vereniging van Tweelingen	Nieuwe Maanderbuurtweg 37, 6717 AN Ede, The Netherlands
Compagnie des Jumelles	19 Rue Melingue, 76019 Paris, France
National Organization of Japan Mothers of Twins Club	Minami-Aoyuma 5-5-21, Minato-Ku, Tokyo, Japan
Foundation for the Study of Infant Deaths	4 Grosvenor Place, London SW1X 7HD, England
The Compassionate Friends	2 Norden Road, Blandford, Dorset DT11 7LT, England
Stillbirth and Perinatal Death Association	15a Christchurch Hill, London NW3, England

References

Aberg, A., Mitelman, F. & Cantz, M. (1978) Cardiac puncture of fetus with Hurler's disease avoiding abortion of unaffected co-twin. *Lancet, ii,* 990–1.

Abraham, J.M., (1967) Intrauterine feto-fetal transfusion syndrome. *Clin. Pediatr., 6,* 405–10.

Abraham, J.M. (1969) Character of placentation in twins, as related to hemoglobin levels. *Clin. Pediatr., 8,* 526–30.

Abrams, R.H. (1957) Double pregnancy. Report of a case with 35 days between deliveries. *Obstet. Gynecol., 9,* 435–8.

Adams, D.L. & Fetterhoff, C.K. (1971) Locked twins. A case report. *Obstet. Gynecol., 38,* 383–5.

Addy, H.L. (1975) The breastfeeding of twins. *J. Trop. Pediatr. Env. Ch. Health, 21,* 231–9.

Adeleye, J.A. (1972) Retained second twin in Ibaden: its fate and management. *Am. J. Obstet. Gynecol., 114,* 204–7.

Aherne, W. & Dunnill, M.S. (1966) Quantitative aspects of placental structure. *J. Path. Bact., 91,* 123–39.

Aherne, W., Strong, S.J. & Corney, G. (1968) The structure cᶠ the placenta in the twin transfusion syndrome. *Biol. Neonat., 12,* 121–35.

Aiken, R.A. (1969) An account of the Birmingham 'sextuplets'. *J. Obstet. Gynaecol. Br. Cwlth., 76,* 684–91.

Alberman, E.D. (1964) Cerebral palsy in twins. *Guys Hospital Report, 133,* 285–95.

Allen, G. (1981) The twinning and fertility paradox. In: *Twin Research 3: Twin Biology and Multiple Pregnancy,* ed. W. Nance, pp. 1–13. New York. Alan R. Liss.

Allen, G. & Kallmann, F.J. (1962) Etiology of mental subnormality in twins. In: *Expanding Goals of Genetics in Psychiatry,* ed. F.J. Kallmann, Chapter 21. London: Grune and Stratton.

Allen, G. & Schachter, J. (1970) Do conception delays explain some changes in twinning rates? *Acta Genet. Med. Gemellol. (Roma) 21,* 30–4.

Allen, G. & Schachter, J. (1971) Ease of conception in mothers of twins. *Soc. Biol. 18,* 18–27.

Allen, J.P. (1972) Twin transfusion syndrome. *Northwest Med. 71,* 296–8.

Allen, M.G., Greenspan, S.I. & Pollin, W. (1976) The effect of parental perceptions on early development in twins. *Psychiatry, 39,* 65–71.

Allen, M.G., Pollin, W. & Hoffer, A. (1971) Parental birth and infancy factors in infant twin development. *Am. J. Psychiatry 127,* 1597–604.

Alm, I. (1953) The long term prognosis for prematurely born children. *Acta Paediatr. 42, Suppl. 94,* 9–116.

Anderson, R.C. (1977) Congenital cardiac malformations in 109 sets of twins and triplets. *Am. J. Cardiol., 39,* 1045–50.

188

Anderson, W.J.R. (1956) Stillbirth and neonatal mortality in twin pregnancy. *J. Obstet. Gynaecol. Br. Emp.*, *63*, 205–15.

Archer, J. (1810) Facts illustrating a disease peculiar to the female children of negro slaves; and observations showing that a white woman by intercourse with a white man and a negro may conceive twins, one of which shall be white and the other a mulatto: and that, vice versa, a black woman by intercourse with a negro and a white man may conceive twins, one of which shall be white and the other a mulatto. *Med. Reposit. N Y*, *1*, 319–23.

Asher, P. & Schonell, F.E. (1950) A survey of 400 cases of cerebral palsy in childhood. *Arch. Dis. Child.*, *25*, 360–79.

Atlay, R.D. & Pennington, G.W. (1971) The use of clomiphene citrate and pituitary gonadotrophin in successive pregnancies. The Sheffield Quadruplets. *Am. J. Obstet. Gynecol.*, *109*, 402–7.

Avery, L.J. (1972) *The Lact-Aid Supplementer*. Denver, Colorado.

Babson, S.G. & Phillips, D.S. (1973) Growth and development of twins dissimilar in size at birth. *N. Engl. J. Med.*, *289*, 937–40.

Barnes, S.E., Bryan, E.M., Harris, D. & Baum, J.D. (1977) Oedema in the newborn. *Molecular Aspects of Medicine*, *1*, No. 3.

Behrman, S.J. (1965) Hazards of twin pregnancies. *Postgrad. Med. 38*, 72–7.

Beischer, N.A., Pepperell, R.J. & Barrie, J.U. (1969) Twin pregnancy and erythroblastosis. *Obstet. Gynecol.*, *34*, 22–9.

Benda, C.E. (1952) Cerebral palsy, birth injuries and anoxia. In: *Developmental Disorders of Mentation and Cerebral Palsies*, Chapter 11, pp. 221–91. New York: Grune and Stratton.

Bender, S. (1952) Twin pregnancy: a review of 472 cases. *J. Obstet. Gynaecol. Br. Emp.*, *59*, 510–7.

Benirschke, K. (1972) Prenatal cardiovascular adaptation. Comparative pathophysiology of circulatory disturbances. In: *Advances in Experimental Medicine and Biology 22*, ed. C.M. Bloor, p. 3. New York: Plenum Press.

Benirschke, K. & Driscoll, S.G. (1967) *The Pathology of the Human Placenta*. New York: Springer-Verlag.

Benirschke, K. & Kim, C.K. (1973) Multiple pregnancy. *N. Engl. J. Med.*, *288*, 1276–84, 1329–36.

Berg, J.M. & Kirman, B.H. (1960) The mentally defective twin. *Br. Med. J.*, *1*, 1911–7.

Bergsma, D. (1967) Conjoined twins. In: *Birth Defects*. Original Article Series 3, No. 1. New York: The National Foundation.

Bernabei, P. & Levi, G. (1976) Psychopathologic problems in twins during childhood. *Acta Genet. Med. Gemellol. (Roma)*, *25*, 381–3.

Bernstein, B.A. (1980) Siblings of twins. *Psychoanal. Study Child 35*, 134–54.

Bessis, R. & Papiernik, E. (1981) Echographic imagery of amniotic membranes in twin pregnancies. In: *Twin Research 3: Twin Biology and Multiple Pregnancy*, ed. W. Nance, pp. 183–7. New York: Alan R. Liss.

Bhargava, I. (1976) Blood vessels of twin placenta in relation to zygosity. *Acta Genet. Med. Gemellol. (Roma)*, *25*, 121–4.

Bhettay, G., Nelson, M.M. & Beighton, P. (1975) Epidemic of conjoined twins in Southern Africa. *Lancet*, *ii*, 741–3.

Blake, A., Stewart, A. & Turcan, D. (1975) Parents of babies of very low birthweight: long-term follow up. In: *Parent–Infant Interaction*, Ciba Foundation Symposium 33, pp. 271–81. Amsterdam: Elsevier.

Bleisch, V.R. (1964) Diagnosis of monochorionic twin placentation. *Am. J. Clin. Pathol.*, *42*, 277–84.

Bluglass, K. (1980) Psychiatric morbidity after cot death. *Practitioner*, *224*, 533–9.

Bosma, J.F. (1954) Autotransfusion between two twins. *Am. J. Dis. Child.*, *88*, 509.

Bourne, G.H. (1962) The human amnion and chorion. London: Lloyd-Luke.

Bourne, S. (1968) The psychological effects of stillbirths on women and their doctors. *J.R. Coll. Gen. Pract.*, *16*, 103–12.

Bowlby, J. (1980) Attachment and Loss, III—Loss sadness and depression. London: Hogarth Press.

Boyd, J.D. & Hamilton, W.J. (1970) *The Human Placenta*. Cambridge: Heffer.

Bracken, M.B. (1979) Oral contraception and twinning: an epidemiologic study. *Am. J. Obstet. Gynecol.*, *133*, 432–4.

Brewster, D.P. (1979) Nursing twins. In: *You can Breastfeed your Baby ... Even in Special Situations*, Chapter 18, pp. 399–414. Emmaus Pa., USA: Rodale Press.

Brock, D.J.H., Barron, L., Watt, M. & Scrimgeour, J.B. (1979) The relation between maternal plasma alphafetoprotein and birthweight in twin pregnancy. *Br. J. Obstet. Gynaecol.*, *86*, 710–12.

Brown, B. (1977) Placentation effects on birth weight in I.Q. in M.Z. twins. Presented to the Society for Research in Child Development, New Orleans.

Bryan, E.M. (1976) Serum immunoglobulins in twin pregnancy with particular reference to the fetofetal transfusion syndrome. M.D. Thesis, London.

Bryan, E.M. (1977*a*) IgG deficiency with placental oedema. *Early Hum. Dev.*, *1*, 133–43.

Bryan, E.M. (1977*b*) Twins are a handful. How can we help? *Maternal and Child Health*, 348–53.

Bryan, E.M. & Kohler, H. (1974) The missing umbilical artery. Prospective study based on a maternity unit. *Arch. Dis. Child.*, *49*, 844–51.

Bryan, E. & Slavin, B. (1974) Serum IgG levels in feto-fetal transfusion syndrome. *Arch. Dis. Child.*, *49*, 908–10.

Bryan, E.M., Slavin, B. & Nicholson, E. (1976) Serum immunoglobulins in multiple pregnancy. *Arch. Dis. Child.*, *51*, 354–9.

Buckler, J.M.H. & Robinson, A. (1974) Matched development of a pair of monozygotic twins of grossly different size at birth. *Arch. Dis. Child.*, *49*, 472–6.

Bulmer, M.G. (1958*a*) The numbers of human multiple births. *Ann. Hum. Genet.*, *22*, 158–64.

Bulmer, M.G. (1958*b*) The repeat frequency of twinning. *Ann. Hum. Genet.*, *23*, 31–5.

Bulmer, M.G. (1959*a*) The effect of parental age, parity and duration of marriage on the twinning rate. *Ann. Hum. Genet.*, *23*, 454–8.

Bulmer, M.G. (1959*b*) Twinning rate in Europe during the war. *Br. Med. J.*, *i*, 29–30.

Bulmer, M.G. (1960) The twinning rate in Europe and Africa. *Ann. Hum. Genet. 24*, 121–5.

Bulmer, M.G. (1970) *The Biology of Twinning in Man*. Oxford: Clarendon Press.

Burlingham, D. (1952) *Twins: a Study of 3 Pairs of Identical Twins*. New York: International Press.

Burnell, G.M. (1974) Maternal reaction to the loss of multiple births. A case of septuplets. *Arch. Gen. Psychiatry*, *30*, 183–4.

Butler, N.R. & Alberman, E.D. (1969) Perinatal problems—the second report of the 1958 British Perinatal Mortality Survey. Edinburgh, London: E. & S. Livingstone.

Cameron, A.H. (1968) The Birmingham twin survey. *Proc. R. Soc. Med.*, *61*, 229–34.

Cameron, A.H., Robson, E.B., Wade-Evans, J. & Wingham, J. (1969) Septuplet conception: placental and zygosity studies. *J. Obstet. Gynaecol. Br. Cwlth.*, *76*, 692–8.

Campbell, D.M., Campbell, A.J. & MacGillivray, I. (1974) Maternal characteristics of women having twin pregnancies. *J. Biosoc. Sci.*, *6*, 463–70.

Campbell, D.M., MacGillivray, I. & Thompson, B. (1977) Twin zygosity and pre-eclampsia. *Lancet*, *ii*, 97 (letter).

Campbell, M. (1961) Twins and congenital heart disease. *Acta Genet. Med. Gemellol. (Roma)*, *10*, 443–55.

Campbell, S. & Dewhurst, C.J. (1970) Quintuplet pregnancy diagnosed and assessed by ultrasonic compound scanning. *Lancet*, *i*, 101–3.

Carpenter, R.G. (1965) Sudden death in twins. *M.O.H. Rep. Publ. Hlth. Med. Subjects, 113*, 51–2.

Carpenter, R.G., Gardner, A., Pursall, E., McWeeney, P.M. & Emery, J.L. (1979) Identification of some infants at immediate risk of dying unexpectedly and justifying intensive study. *Lancet*, *ii*, 343–6.

Carter, C.O. (1965) The inheritance of common congenital malformations. In: *Progress in Medical Genetics 4*, ed. A.G. Steinberg & A.G. Bearn, pp. 59–84. London: Heineman.

Cederlof, R., Friberg, L., Jonsson, E. & Kaij, L. (1961) Studies on similarity diagnosis in twins with the aid of mailed questionnaires. *Acta Genet.*, *11*, 338–62.

Chamberlain, R.N. & Simpson, R.N. (1977) Cross-sectional studies of physical growth in twins, postmature and small-for-dates children. *Acta Pediatr. Scand.*, *66*, 457–63.

Christoffel, K.K. & Salafsky, I. (1975) Fetal alcohol syndrome in dizygotic twins. *J. Pediatr.*, *87*, 963–7.

Churchill, J.A. & Henderson, W. (1974) Perinatal factors affecting fetal development—twin pregnancy. In: *Birth Defects and Fetal Development*, ed. K.S. Moghissi, Chapter 4, pp. 69–76. Springfield, Ill.: Charles C. Thomas.

Clemetson, C.A.B. (1956) The difference in birthweight in human twins. 2. Cord blood haemoglobin levels. *J. Obstet. Gynaecol. Br. Emp.*, *63*, 9–14.

Cohen, D.J., Dibble, E., Grawe, J.M. & Pollin, W. (1975). Reliably separating identical from fraternal twins. *Arch. Gen. Psychiatry 32*, 1371–5.

Cooke, R.T. & Welch, R.G. (1964) A study in cot death. *Br. Med. J.*, *2*, 1549–54.

Corey, L.A., Nance, W.E., Kang, K.W. & Christian, J.C. (1979) Effects of type of placentation on birth weight and its variability in monozygotic and dizygotic twins. *Acta Genet. Med. Gemellol. (Roma)*, *28*, 41–50.

Corney, G. (1966) The Twin Transfusion Syndrome. M.D. Thesis (University of Liverpool).

Corney, G. (1975*a*) Mythology and customs associated with twins. In: *Human Multiple Reproduction*, MacGillivray, I., Nylander, P.P.S. & Corney, G., Chapter I, pp. 1–15. London: W.B. Saunders.

Corney, G. (1975*b*) Placentation. In: *Human Multiple Reproduction*, MacGillivray, I., Nylander, P.P.S. & Corney, G., Chapter 3, pp. 40–76. London: W.B. Saunders.

Corney, G. & Robson, E.B. (1975) Types of twinning and determination of zygosity. In: *Human Multiple Reproduction*, MacGillivray, I., Nylander, P.P.S. & Corney, G.,Chapter 2, pp. 16–39. London: W.B. Saunders.

Corney, G., Robson, E.B. & Strong, S.J. (1972) The effect of zygosity on the birth weight of twins. *Ann. Hum. Genet.*, *36*, 45–59.

Corney, G., Seedburgh, D., Thompson, B., Campbell, D.M., MacGillivray, I. & Timlin, D. (1979) Maternal height and twinning. *Ann. Hum. Genet.*, *43*, 55–9.

Corston, J. McD. (1957) Twin survival. A comparison of mortality rates of the first and second twin. *Obstet. Gynaecol. 10*, 181–3.

Cortes, R.L. (1964) Cuadruples con transfusion de feto a feto un producto con anemia y otro con policitemia. *Revista Medica de Costa Rica*, *21*, 89–99.

Cotton, M., Cotton, G. & Goodall, J. (1981) A brother dies at home. *Maternal and Child Health*, *6*, 288–92.

Cox, M.L. (1963) Incidence and aetiology of multiple births in Nigeria. *J. Obstet. Gynaecol. Br. Cwlth.*, *70*, 878–84.

Crane, J.P., Tomich, P.G. & Kopta, M. (1980) Ultrasonic growth patterns and discordant twins. *Obstet. Gynecol. 55*, 678–83.

Curtius, F. (1928) Quoted by M.G. Bulmer in *The Biology of Twinning in Man* (1970). Oxford: Clarendon Press.

Czeizel, A. & Acsádi, G. (1971) Demographic characteristics of multiple births in Hungary. *Acta Genet. Med. Gemellol (Roma)*, *20*, 301–13.

Dahlberg, G. (1926) *Twin Births and Twins from a Hereditary Point of View*. Stockholm: A.B. Tidens Tryckeri.

Danielson, C. (1960) Twin pregnancy and birth. *Acta Obstet. Gynecol.*, *39*, 63–87.

Davenport, C.B. (1927) Does the male have an influence in human twin production? *Zeitschrift für induktiv Abstammungs and Vererbungslehre*, *46*, 85–6.

Davis, E.A. (1937) Linguistic skill in twins, singletons and siblings and only children from age five to ten years. *Univ. Minn. Instit. Child Welfare Monogr. Series No. 14*.

Dawood, M.Y., Ratnam, S.S. & Lim, Y.C. (1975) Twin pregnancy in Singapore. *Aust. N.Z. J. Obstet. Gynaecol.*, *15*, 93–8.

Day, E. (1932) The development of language in twins. I. A comparison of twins and single children. *Child Dev.*, *3*, 179–99.

Divers, W.A. & Hemsell, D.L. (1979) The use of ultrasound in multiple gestations. *Obstet. Gynecol. 53*, 500–4.

Dorgan, L.T. & Clarke, P.E. (1956) Uterus didelphys with double pregnancy. *Am. J. Obstet. Gynecol.*, 72, 663–6.

Douglas, B. (1958) The role of environmental factors in the etiology of 'so-called' congenital malformations I & II. *Plast. Reconstr. Surg.*, 22, 94–108, 214–29.

Douglas, J.E. & Sutton, A. (1978) The development of speech and mental processes in a pair of twins: A case study. *Child Psychol. Psychiat.*, 19, 49–56.

Drillien, C.M. (1964) *The Growth and Development of the Prematurely Born Infant.* Baltimore, Md: Williams and Wilkins Co.

Drucker, P., Finkel, J. & Savel, L.E. (1960) Sixty-five day interval between the births of twins. A case report. *Am. J. Obstet. Gynecol.*, 80, 761–3.

Dubowitz, L.M.S., Dubowitz, V. & Goldberg, C. (1970) Clinical assessment of gestational age in the newborn infant. *J. Pediatr.*, 77, 1–10.

Dunn, P. (1965) Some perinatal observations on twins. *Dev. Med. Ch. Neurol.*, 7, 121–34.

Durkin, M.V., Kaveggia, E.G., Pendleton, E., Neuhauser, G. & Opitz, J.M. (1976) Analysis of etiologic factors in cerebral palsy with severe mental retardation. 1. Analysis of gestational, parturitional and neonatal data. *Eur. J. Pediatr.*, 123, 67–81.

Eastman, N.J. (1961) Editorial comments. *Obstet. Gynecol. Survey 16*, 185.

Eastman, N.J., Kohl, S.G., Maisel, J.E. & Kavaler, F. (1962) The obstetrical background of 753 cases of cerebal palsy. *Obstet. Gynecol. Survey*, 17, 459–97.

Editorial (1976) Koluchova's twins. *Br. Med. J.*, 897–8.

Editorial (1977) Preventing prematurity in twins. *Br. Med. J.*, i, 1618.

Edmonds, H.W., (1954) The spiral of the normal umbilical cord in twins and in singletons. *Am. J. Obstet. Gynecol.*, 67, 102–20.

Edwards, J. (1938) Season and rate of conception. *Nature (Lond)*, 142, 357.

Elias, S., Gerbie, A.B., Simpson, J.L., Nadler, H.L., Sabbagha, R.E. & Shkolnik, A. (1980) Genetic amniocentesis in twin gestations. *Am. J. Obstet. Gynecol.*, 138, 169–74.

Ellis, R.F., Berger, G.S., Keith, L. & Depp, R. (1979) The North Western University multi hospital twin study. II Mortality of first versus second twins. *Acta. Genet. Med. Gemollol. (Roma)*, 28, 347–52.

Elwood, J.M., (1973) Changes in the twinning rate in Canada 1926–1970. *Br. J. Prev. Soc. Med.* 27, 236–41.

Elwood, J.M., (1978) Maternal and environmental factors affecting twin births in Canadian cities. *Br. J. Obstet. Gynaecol.*, 85, 351–8.

Emery, J.L., (1979) Cot death. *Maternal and Child Health*, 4, 374–8.

Eriksson, A.W. & Fellman, J. (1967) Twinning in relation to the marital status of the mother. *Acta Genet.*, 17, 385–98.

Eriksson, A.W. & Fellman, J.O. (1973) Differences in the twinning trends between Finns and Swedes. *Am. J. Hum. Genet.*, 25, 141–51.

Eriksson, A.W., Eskola, M.R. & Fellman, J.O., (1976) Retrospective studies on the twinning rate in Scandinavia. *Acta Genet. Med. Gemollol. (Roma)*, 25, 29–35.

Falkner, F. (1978) Implications for growth in human twins. In: *Human Growth 1 Principles and Prenatal Growth*, ed. F. Falkner and J.M. Tanner, Chapter 16, pp. 397–413. London: Baillière Tindall.

Farooqui, M.O., Grossman, J.H. & Shannon, R.A. (1973) A review of twin pregnancy and perinatal mortality. *Obstet. Gynecol. Survey.*, 28, 144–53.

Farr, V. (1975) Prognosis for the babies, early and late. In: *Human Multiple Reproduction*, MacGillivray, I., Nylander, P.P.S. & Corney, G., Chapter 14, pp. 188–211. London: W.B. Saunders.

Farrell, A.G.W. (1964) Twin Pregnancy: a study of 1,000 cases. *S. Afr. J. Obstet. Gynaecol.*, 2, 35–41.

Fenner, A., Malm, T. & Kurrerow, U. (1980) Intrauterine growth of twins. A retrospective analysis. *Eur. J. Pediatr.*, 133, 119–21.

Ferguson, W.F. (1964) Perinatal mortality in multiple gestations. A review of perinatal deaths from 1609 multiple gestations. *Obstet. Gynecol.*, 23, 861–70.

Field, T. & Widmayer, S. (1980) Early development of term and preterm twins. University of Miami Medical School. Paper presented at New Haven.

Finberg, H.J. & Birnholz, J.C. (1979) Ultrasound observations in multiple gestation with first trimester bleeding: the blighted twin. *Radiology*, *132*, 137–42.

Foglmann, R. (1976) Monoamniotic twins. *Acta Genet. Med. Gemellol (Roma)*, *26*, 62–5.

Forrester, R.M., Lees, V.T. & Watson, G.H. (1966) Rubella syndrome: escape of a twin. *Br. Med. J.*, *1*, 1403.

Fox, H. (1978) The Placenta in Multiple Pregnancy In: *Pathology of the Placenta*, Chapter 4, pp. 73–94. London: W.B. Saunders.

Friedman, E.A. & Sachtleben, M.R. (1964) The effect of uterine distension in labor. Multiple pregnancy. *Obstet. Gynecol.*, *23*, 164–72.

Froggatt, P., Lynas, M.A. & McKenzie, G. (1971) Epidemiology of sudden unexpected death in infants ('cot death') in Northern Ireland. *Br. J. Prev. Soc. Med.*, *25*, 119–34.

Fujikura, T. & Froehlich, L.A. (1971) Twin placentation and zygosity. *Obstet. Gynecol.*, *37*, 34–43.

Fujikura, T. & Froehlich, L. (1974) Mental and motor development in monozygotic co-twins with dissimilar birth weights. *Pediatrics*, *53*, 884–9.

Garrett, W.J. (1960) Uterine overdistension and the duration of labour. *Med. J. Aust.*, *2*, 376–7.

Gedda, L. (1961) *Twins in History and Science*. Springfield, Ill.: Charles C. Thomas.

Geyer, E. (1940) Ein Zwillingspärchen mit zwei Vätern (nachgewiesne Überschwängerung beim Menschen). *Arch. Rassenbiol.*, *34*, 226–36.

Gifford, S., Murawski, B.J. & Brazelton, T.B. (1966) Differences in individual development within a pair of identical twins. *Int. J. Psychoanal.*, *47*, 261–8.

Giovannucci-Uzielli, M.L., Vecchi, C., Donzelli, G.P. & Levi d'Ancona Lepi, E. (1981) The history of the Florentine sextuplets: obstetric and genetic considerations. *Twin Research 3 Twin Biology and Multiple Pregnancy*, ed. W. Nance, pp. 217–20. New York: Alan R. Liss.

Goldgar, D.E. & Kimberling, W.J. (1981) Genetic expectations of polar body twinning. *Acta Genet. Med. Gemellol. 30*, 257–66.

Goplerud, C.P. (1964) Monoamniotic twins with double survival. *Obstet. Gynecol.*, *23*, 289–90.

Goshen-Gottstein, E. (1980) The mothering of twins, triplets and quadruplets. *Psychiatry*, *43*, 189–204.

Grant, P. & Pearn, J.H. (1969) Foetus-in-foetu. *Med. J. Aust.*, 1016-9.

Green, Q.L., Schanck, G.P. & Smith, J.R. (1961) Normal, living twins in uterus didelphys with 38 day interval between deliveries. *Am. J. Obstet. Gynecol*, *82*, 340–2.

Greenspan, L. & Deaver, G.G. (1953) Clinical approach to the etiology of cerebral palsy. *Arch. Phys. Med. Rehab.*, *34*, 478–85.

Grennert, L., Persson, P.H., Gennser, G., Kullander, S. & Thorelli, J. (1976) Ultrasound and human-placental-lactogen screening for early detection of twin pregnancies. *Lancet*, *i*, 4–6.

Greulich, W.W. (1934) Heredity in human twinning. *Am. J. Phys. Anthropol.*, *19*, 391–431.

Griffiths, M. (1967) Cerebral palsy in multiple pregnancy. *Dev. Med. Child Neurol.*, *9*, 713–31.

Griffiths, M.I. (1981) The hospital treatment of twins in childhood. In: *Twins Research (Birmingham 1968–72) Vol. 2*, ed. C.J. Phillips Part IV, pp. 225–41. Centre for Child Study, University of Birmingham.

Gross, R.E., Clatworthy, H.W. & Mecker, J.A. (1951) Sacrococcygeal teratomas in infants and children. *Surg. Gynecol.*, *92*, 341–54.

Gruenwald, P. (1970) Environmental influences on twins apparent at birth: a preliminary study. *Biol. Neonat.*, *15*, 79–93.

Gunther, M. (1973) *Infant Feeding*. London: Penguin Books.

Guttmacher, A.F. (1939) An analysis of 573 cases of twin pregnancy. *Am. J. Obstet. Gynecol.*, *38*, 277–88.

Guttmacher, A.F. & Kohl, S.G. (1958) The fetus of multiple gestations. *Obstet. Gynecol.*, *12*, 528–41.

Guttmacher, A.F. & Nichols, B.L. (1967) Teratology of conjoined twins. In: Conjoined Twins, ed. D. Bergsma, pp. 3–7. *Birth Defects. Original Article Series*, *3*, No. 1.

Hamon, A. & Dinno, N. (1978) Dicephalus dipus tribrachius conjoined twins in a female infant. *Birth Defects*, *14*, 213–8.

Hanson, J.W. (1975) Incidence of conjoined twinning. *Lancet ii*, 1957.

Harvey, M.A.S., Huntley, R.M.C. & Smith, D.W. (1977) Familial monozygotic twinning. *J. Pediatr.*, *90*, 246–7.

Hay, S. & Wehrung, D.A. (1970) Congenital malformations in twins. *Am. J. Hum. Genet.*, *22*, 662–78.

Heady, J.A. & Heasman, M.A. (1955) *Social and biological factors in infant mortality*. General Register Office, Studies on medical and population subjects 15. London H.M.S.O.

Hellin, D. (1895) *Die Ursache der Multiparität der unipaaren Tiere überhaupt und der Zwillingsschwangerschaft beim Menschen insbesondere*. München.

Hemon, D., Berger, C. & Lazar, P. (1979) The etiology of human dizygotic twinning with special reference to spontaneous abortions. *Acta Genet. Med. Gemollol (Roma) 28*, 253–8.

Hemon, D., Berger, C. & Lazar, P., (1982) Interaction between twinning and maternal factors associated with small for dateness. Presented at the International Workshop on Twins, Paris.

Hendricks, C.H. (1966) Twinning in relation to birth weight, mortality and congenital anomalies. *Obstet. Gynecol.*, *27*, 47–53.

Henriksen, J.B., Flugsrud, L.B. & Orstavik, I. (1968) Cytomegali hos en nyfødt tvilling påvist ved isolation av cytomegalvirus. *Tidsskr. Nor. Laegeforen.*, *88*, 81.

Herlitz, G. (1941) Zur Kenntnis der anämischen und polyzytämischen Zustande bei Neugenborenensowie des Icterus gravis neonatorum. *Acta Paediatr.*, *29*, 211–53.

Hewitt, D. & Stewart, A. (1970) Relevance of twin data to intrauterine selection. *Acta Genet. Med. Gemollol (Roma) 19*, 83–6.

Hibbard, B.M. (1959) Hydrops foetalis in one of uniovular twins. *J. Obstet. Gynaecol. Br. Emp.*, *66*, 649–53.

Hoefnagel, D. & Benirschke, K. (1962) Twinning in Klinefelter's Syndrome. *Lancet, ii*, 1282.

Hoffman, H.J., Bakketeig, L.S. & Stark, C.R. (1978) Twins and perinatal mortality: a comparison between single and twin births in Minnesota and in Norway. 1967–73. *Prog. Clin. Biol. Res.*, *246*, 133–42.

Holt, S.B. (1968) *The Genetics of Dermal Ridges*. Springfield, Ill.: Charles C. Thomas.

Hunter, A.G. & Cox, D.M. (1979) Counselling problems when twins are discovered at genetic amniocentesis. *Clin. Genet.*, *16*, 34–42.

Husén, T. (1959) *Psychological Twin Research*. Stockholm: Almquist and Wiksell.

Husén, T. (1961) Abilities of twins. *Acta Psychol.*, *19*, 1–2.

Husén, T. (1963) Intra-pair similarities in the school achievements of twins. *Scand. J. Psychol.*, *4*, 108–14.

Hyrtl, J. (1870) Die Blutgefässe der menschlichen Nachgeburt. Vienna: W. Braumüller.

Idelberger, K. (1929) Die Zwillings pathologie des angeborenen Klumpfuss. Beilagehft zur *Zeitschrift für Ornithologie und praktische Geflügelzucht*, *69*.

Idelberger, K. (1951) *Der Erb pathologie der Segamaunter angeborenen Heift Vervenkung.* München, Berlin: Urban and Schwarzenburg.

Inouye, E. & Imaizumi, Y. (1981) Analysis of twinning rates in Japan. *Twin Research 3 Twin Biology and Multiple Pregnancy*, ed. W. Nance, pp. 21–33. New York: Alan R. Liss.

Jackson, E.W., Norris, F.D. & Kauber, M.R. (1969) Childhood leukaemia in California-born twins. *Cancer*, *23*, 913–9.

James, F.M., Crawford, J.S., Davies, P. & Naiem, H. (1977) Lumbar epidural analgesia for labor and delivery of twins. *Am. J. Obstet. Gynecol. 127*, 176–80.

James, W.H. (1972a) Coital rates and dizygotic twinning. *J. Biosoc. Sci.*, *4*, 101–5.

James, W.H. (1972b) Secular changes in dizygotic twinning rates. *J. Biosoc. Sci.*, *4*, 427–34.

James, W.H. (1975) The secular decline in dizygotic twinning rates in Italy. *Acta Genet. Med. Gemellol (Roma)*, *24*, 9–14.

James, W.H. (1977) The sex ratio of monoamniotic twin pairs. *Ann. Hum. Biol.*, *4*, 143–53.

James, W.H. (1978) A hypothesis on the declining dizygotic twinning rates in developed countries. *Prog. Clin. Biol. Res.*, *24*, 81–8.

Janovski, N.A. (1962) Fetus in fetu. *J. Pediatr. 61*, 100–4.

Jarvis, G.J. (1979) Diagnosis of multiple pregnancy. *Br. Med. J.*, *2*, 593–4.

Jaschevatzky, O.E., Shalit, A., Levy, Y. & Grunstein, S. (1977) Epidural analgesia during labour in twin pregnancy. *Br. J. Obstet. Gynaecol.*, *84*, 327–31.

Jassani, M.N., Merkatz, I.R., Brennan, J.N. & MacIntyre, M.N. (1980) Twin pregnancy with discordancy for Down's syndrome. *Obstet. Gynecol.*, *55*, Suppl. 455–65.

Javert, C.T. (1957) *Spontaneous and Habitual Abortion*. New York: Blakiston.

Jeanneret, O. & MacMahon, B. (1962) Secular changes in rates of multiple births in the United States. *Am. J. Hum. Genet. 14*, 410–25.

Jeffreys, M.D.W. (1953) Twin births among Africans. *S. Afr. J. Sci.*, *50*, 89–93.

Jelliffe, D.B. & Jelliffe, E.F.P. (1975) Human milk, nutrition and the world resource crisis. *Science (NY)*, *188*, 557–61.

Jelliffe, D.B. & Jelliffe, E.F.P. (1978) *Human Milk in the Modern World. (Psychosocial, Nutritional, and Economic Significance)*. Oxford University Press.

Jewelewicz, R., James, S.L., Finster, M., Dyrenfurth, I., Warren, M.P. & Wiele, R.L.V. (1972) Quintuplet gestation after ovulation induction with menopausal gonadotropins and pituitary luteinising hormone. *Obstet. Gynecol.*, *40*, 1–5.

Jorgensen, G., Bettren, A.J., Stoermer, J. (1971) Genetische Untersuchungen bei verschiedenen Typen angeborener Herzfehler. *Mschr. Kinderhelk*, *119*, 417–21.

Jovanovic, L., Landesman, R. & Saxena, B.B. (1977) Screening for twin pregnancy. *Science, 198*, 738.

Kaelber, C.T. & Pugh, T.F. (1969) Influence of intrauterine relations on the intelligence of twins. *N. Engl. J. Med.*, *280*, 1030–4.

Kamimura, K. (1976) Epidemiology of twin births from a climatic point of view. *Br. J. Prev. Soc. Med.*, *30*, 175–9.

Karn, M.N. & Penrose, L.S. (1952) Birth weight and length of gestation of twins together with maternal age, parity and survival rate. *Ann. Eugen.*, *16*, 365–77.

Kasriel, J. & Eaves, L. (1976) The zygosity of twins, further evidence of the agreement between diagnosis by blood groups and written questionnaires. *J. Biosoc. Sci.*, *8*, 263–6.

Kauppila, A., Joupila, P., Koivisto, M., Moilanen, I. & Ylikorkala, O. (1975) Twin Pregnancy. A clinical study of 335 cases. *Acta Obstet. Gynecol. Scand. Suppl.* 44, 5–12.

Keay, A.J. (1958) The significance of twins in mongolism in the light of new evidence. *J. Ment. Defic. Res.*, *2*, 1–7.

Keet, M.P., Jaroszewicz, A.M. & Liebenberg, A. Le R. (1974) Assessment of gestational age in twins. *Arch. Dis. Child.*, *49*, 741–2.

Kenna, A.P., Smithells, R.W. & Fielding, D.W. (1975) Congenital heart disease in Liverpool: 1960–69. *Q. J. Med.*, *154*, 17–44.

Kennell, J.H., Klaus, M.H., Sosa, R. & Urrutia, J. (1976) Early neonatal contact: effect on growth breastfeeding and infection in the first year of life. *Pediatr. Res.*, *10*, 426.

Kerenyi, T.D. & Chitkara, U. (1981) Selective birth in twin pregnancy with discordancy for Down's syndrome. *N. Engl. J. Med.*, *304*, 1525–7.

Kerr, M.G. & Rashad, M.N. (1966) Autosomal trisomy in a discordant monozygotic twin. *Nature (Lond.)*, *212*, 726–7.

Khoo, S.K. & Green, K. (1975) Twin pregnancies, influence of antenatal complications, hospital bed rest, and misdiagnosis on prematurity and perinatal mortality. *Aust. N.Z. J. Obstet. Gynecol.*, *15*, 84–92.

Khunda, S. (1972) Locked Twins. *Obstet. Gynecol.*, *39*, 453–9.

Kim, C.C., Dales, R.J., Connor, R., Walters, J. & Witherspoon, R. (1969) Social interaction of like-sex twins and singletons in relation to intelligence, language and physical development. *J. Genet. Psychol.*, *114*, 203–14.

Kindred, J.E. (1944) Twin pregnancies with one twin blighted. *Am. J. Obstet. Gynecol.*, *48*, 642–82.

Klaus, M.H. & Kennell, J.H. (1970) Mothers separated from their newborn infants. *Pediatr. Clin. North Am.*, *17*, 1015–37.

Klaus, M.H., Kennell, J.H., Plumb, N. & Zuehlke, S. (1970) Human maternal behaviour at the first contact with her young. *Pediatrics, 46*, 187–92.

Klebe, J.G. & Ingomar, C.J. (1972) The fetoplacental circulation during parturition illustrated by the interfetal transfusion syndrome. *Pediatrics 49*, 112–6.

Klingberg, W.G., Jones, B., Allen, W.M. & Dempsey, E. (1955) Placental parabiotic circulation of single ovum human twins. *Am. J. Dis. Child.*, *90*, 519–20.

Kloosterman, G.J. (1963) The "third circulation" in identical twins. *Ned. Tijdschr. Verloskd. Gynaecol. 63*, 395–412.

Knight, G.J., Kloza, E.M., Smith, D.E. & Haddow, J.E. (1981) Efficiency of human placental lactogen and alpha-fetoprotein measurement in twin pregnancy detection. *Am. J. Obstet. Gynecol.*, *141*, 585–6.

Knox, E.G. (1970) Fetus–fetus interaction—a model aetiology for anencephalus. *Dev. Med. Child Neurol.*, *12*, 167–77.

Knox, E.G. (1974) Twins and neural tube defects. *Br. J. Prev. Soc. Med.*, *28*, 73–80.

Knox, G. & Morley, D. (1960) Twinning in Yoruba women. *J. Obstet. Gynaecol. Br. Cwlth.*, *67*, 981–4.

Koch, H.L. (1966) *Twins and Twin Relations.* Chicago: University of Chicago Press.

Koivisto, M., Jouppila, P., Kauppila, A., Moilanen, I. & Ylikorkala, O. (1975) Twin pregnancy. Neonatal morbidity and mortality. *Acta Obstet. Gynecol. Scand. Suppl.*, *44*, 21–9.

Koluchova, J. (1972) Severe deprivation of twins: a case study. *J. Child. Psychol. Psychiatry*, *13*, 107–14.

Koluchova, J. (1976) The further development of twins after severe and prolonged deprivation: a second report. *J. Child. Psychol. Psychiatry*, *17*, 181–8.

Korányi, G. & Kovács, J. (1975) Über das Zwillingstransfusionsyndrom. *Acta Paediatr. Acad. Sci. Hung.*, *16*, 119–25.

Kranitz, M.A. & Welcher, D.W. (1971) Behavioural characteristics of twins. *J. Hopkins Med. J.*, *129*, 1–5.

Kraus, J.F. & Borhani, N.O. (1972) Post-neonatal sudden unexplained death in California: a cohort study. *Am. J. Epidemiol.*, *95*, 497–510.

Kristofferson, K. (1969) The significance of absence of one umbilical artery. *Acta Obstet. Gynecol. Scand.*, *48*, 195–214.

Lachelin, G.C.L., Brant, H.A., Swyer, G.I.M., Little, V. & Reynolds, E.O.R. (1972) Sextuplet pregnancy. *Br. Med. J.*, *1*, 787–90.

Laursen, B. (1973) Twin pregnancy. The value of prophylactic rest in bed and the risk involved. *Acta Obstet. Gynecol. Scand.*, *52*, 367–71.

Law, R.G. (1967) *Standards of Obstetric Care: the report of the West Metropolitan Regional Obstetric Survey. 1962–64*, Part II, pp. 92–204. Edinburgh, London: E & S Livingstone.

Layde, P.M., Erickson, J.D., Falek, A. & McCarthy, B.J. (1980) Congenital malformations in twins. *Am. J. Hum. Genet.*, *32*, 69–78.

Lazar, P., Berger, C. & Hemon, D. (1981) Preconceptional prediction of twin pregnancies. In: *Twin Research 3. Twin Biology and Multiple Pregnancy*, ed. W. Nance, pp. 175–81. New York: Alan R. Liss.

Lee, D.A. (1979) Munchausen syndrome by proxy in twins. *Arch. Dis. Child.*, *54*, 646–7.

Le Marec, B., Roussey, M., Oger, J. & Senecal, J. (1978) Excess twinning in the parents of spina bifida. *Prog. Clin. Biol. Res.*, *24b*, 121–3.

Lenz, W. (1966) Malformations caused by drugs in pregnancy. *Am. J. Dis. Child.*, *112*, 99–106.

Leonard, M.R. (1959) Problems in identification and ego development in twins. Presented to American Psychoanalytic Association in Philadelphia.

Leroy, B., Lefort, F. & Jeny, R. (1982) Uterine height and umbilical perimeter curves in twin pregnancies. Presented at the International Workshop on Twin Pregnancies, Paris.

Leveno, K.J., Santos-Ramos, R., Duenhoelter, J.H., Reisch, J.S. & Whalley, P.J. (1979) Sonar cephalometry in twins: a table of biparietal diameters for normal twin fetuses and a comparison with singletons. *Am. J. Obstet. Gynecol.*, *135*, 727–30.

Levi, S. (1976) Ultrasonic assessment of the high rate of human multiple pregnancy in the first trimester. *J. Clin. Ultrasound*, *4*, 3–5.

Lewis, E. (1979a) Inhibition of mourning by pregnancy: psychopathology and management. *Br. Med. J.*, *2*, 27–8.

Lewis, E. (1979b) Mourning by the family after a stillbirth or neonatal death. *Arch. Dis. Child.*, *54*, 303–6.

Lewis, E. (1983) Stillbirth: Psychological consequences and strategies of management. In *Advances in Perinatal Medicine*, 3, ed. A. Mulinsky, E.A. Friedman & I. Gluck. New York: Plenum.

Lewis, E. & Page, A. (1978) Failure to mourn a stillbirth: an overlooked catastrophe. *Br. J. Med. Psychol.*, *51*, 237–41.

Liggins, G.C. & Ibbertson, H.K. (1966) A successful quintuplet pregnancy following treatment with human pituitary gonadotrophin. *Lancet*, *i*, 114–7.

Linney, J. (1980a) The emotional and social aspects of having twins. *Nursing Times*, *76*, 276–79.

Linney, J. (1980b) *Guide for Mothers of Twins*. U.K.: Twins Clubs Association.

Linney, J. (1983) *The Management of Multiple Births*. Wiley: Chichester.

Livingston, J.E. & Poland, B.J. (1980) A study of spontaneously aborted twins. *Teratology*, *21*, 139–48.

Ljung, B.O., Fischbein, S. & Lindgren, G. (1977) Comparison of growth in twins and singleton controls of matched age longitudinally from 10 to 18 years. *Ann. Hum. Biol.*, *4*, 405–15.

Loehlin, J.C. & Nichols, R.C. (1976) *Heredity, Environment and Personality: a study of 850 sets of twins*. Austin: University of Texas Press.

Loughnan, P.M., Gold, H. & Vance, J.C. (1973) Phenytoin teratogenicity in man. *Lancet*, *i*, 70–2.

Lytton, H. (1980) *Parent–Child Interaction. The Socialization Process Observed in Twin and Singleton Families*. New York: Plenum Press.

Lytton, H. & Conway, D. (1977) The impact of twinship on parent–child interaction. *J. Pers. Soc. Psychol.*, *35*, 97–107.

Macafee, C.A.J., Fortune, D.W. & Beischer, N.A. (1970) Non-immunological hydropsfetalis. *J. Obstet. Gynaecol. Br. Cwlth.*, *77*, 226–37.

McArthur, J.W. (1938) Genetics of quintuplets. 1. Diagnosis of the Dionne quintuplets as a monozygotic set. *J. Hered.*, *29*, 323–9.

MacDonald, A.D. (1964) Mongolism in twins. *J. Med. Genet.*, *1*, 39–41.

MacGillivray, I. (1958) Some observations on the incidence of preeclampsia. *J. Obstet. Gynaecol. Br. Emp.*, *65*, 535–9.

MacGillivray, I. (1975a) Diagnosis of twin pregnancy. In: *Human Multiple Reproduction*, MacGillivray, I., Nylander, P.P.S. & Corney, G., Chapter 8, pp. 116–23. London: W.B. Saunders.

MacGillivray, I. (1975b) Labour in multiple pregnancies. In: *Human Multiple Reproduction*, Chapter 11, pp. 147–64. London: W.B. Saunders.

MacGillivray, I. (1975c) Management of multiple pregnancies. In: *Human Multiple Reproduction*, MacGillivray, I., Nylander, P.P.S. & Corney, G., Chapter 9, pp. 124–36. London: W.B. Saunders.

MacGillivray, I. (1982) Preterm labour in twin pregnancies. Presented at the International Workshop on Twin Pregnancies, Paris.

MacGillivray, I., Nylander, P.P.S. & Corney, G. (1975) *Human Multiple Reproduction*. London: W.B. Saunders.

McKeown, T. & Record, R.G. (1952) Observations on foetal growth in multiple pregnancy in man. *J. Endocrinol.*, *8*, 386–401.

McKeown, T. & Record, R.G. (1953) The influence of placental size on foetal growth in man, with special reference to multiple pregnancy. *J. Endocrinol.*, *9*, 418–26.

McKeown, T. & Record, R.G. (1960) Malformations in a population observed for five years. *CIBA Foundation Symposium on Congenital Malformations*, pp. 2–21. London: Churchill.

McManus, I.C. (1980) Handedness in twins. A critical review. *Neuropsychologia*, *18*, 347–55.

Mägiste, M., Von Schenck, H., Sjöberg, N., Thorell, J.I. & Aberg, A. (1976) Screening for detecting twin pregnancy. *Am. J. Obstet. Gynecol.*, *126*, 697–8.

Mannino, F.L., Jones, K.L. & Benirschke, K. (1977) Congenital skin defects and fetus papyraceus, *J. Pediatr.*, *91*, 559–64.

Matheny, A.P. Jr. & Brown, A.M. (1971) The behaviour of twins: effects of birth weight and birth sequence. *Child. Dev.*, *42*, 251–7.

Matheny, A.P., Brown, A.M. & Wilson, R.S. (1971) Behavioural antecedents of accidental injuries in early childhood: a study of twins. *J. Pediatr., 79*, 122–4.

Matheny, A.P., Wilson, R.S. & Dolan, A.B. (1976) Relations between twins' similarity of appearance and behavioural similarity: testing an assumption. *Behav. Genet., 6*, 343–51.

Mauriceau, F. (1721) *Traité des maladies des femmes grosses.* Paris.

Mayer, C.F. (1952a) Sextuplets and higher multiparous births. Part 1, Multiparity and sextuplets. *Acta Genet. Med. Gemellol, (Roma), 1*, 118–35.

Mayer, C.F. (1952b) Sextuplets and higher multiparous births. Part 2: Sextuplets and higher births. *Acta Genet. Med. Gemellol (Roma), 1*, 242–75.

Mead, M. (1957) Changing patterns of parent–child relations in an urban culture. *Int. J. Psychoanal., 38*, 369–78.

Meadow, R. (1977) Munchausen syndrome by proxy—the hinterland of child abuse. *Lancet, ii*, 343–5.

Mehrotra, S.N. & Maxwell, J. (1949) The intelligence of twins: a comparative study of eleven year old twins. *Pop. Stud., 3*, 295–302.

Mellin, G.N. & Katzenstein, M. (1962) The saga of thalidomide. *N. Engl. J. Med., 267*, 1184–93, 1238–44.

Melnick, M. (1977) Brain damage in survivor after death of monozygotic co-twin. *Lancet, ii*, 1287.

Melnick, M. & Myrianthopoulos, N.C. (1979) The effects of chorion type on normal and abnormal developmental variation in monozygous twins. *Am. J. Med. Genet., 4*, 147–56.

Merkatz, I.R. (1979) In: *Care of the High Risk Neonate*, ed. M.H. Klaus & A.A. Faharoff, p. 71. London: W.B. Saunders.

Merrell, Pharmaceuticals Ltd. (1981) Clomid. In: *Data Sheet Compendium*, p. 770. London: Datapharm Publ.

Metrakos, J.D., Metrakos, K. & Baxter, H. (1958) Clefts of the lip and palate in twins, including a discordant pair whose monozygosity was confirmed by skin transplants. *Plast. Reconstr. Surg., 22*, 109–22.

Meyer, W.C., Keith, L. & Webster, A. (1970) Monoamniotic twin pregnancy with the transfusion syndrome. *Chicago Med. Sch. Q., 29*, 42–51.

Michaels, L. (1967) Unilateral ischaemia of the fused twin placenta: a manifestation of the twin transfusion syndrome. *Can. Med. Assoc. J., 96*, 402–5.

Michels, V.V. & Riccardi, V.M. (1978) Twin recurrence and amniocentesis: male and MZ heritability factors. *Birth Defects, 14*, 201–11.

Miettinen, M. (1954) On triplets and quadruplets in Finland. *Acta Paediatr., 43*, Suppl. 99, 9–103.

Miettinen, M. & Grönroos, J.A. (1965) A follow-up study of Finnish Triplets. *Ann. Paediatr. Fenniae. (Helsinki), 11*, 71–83.

Mijsberg, W.A. (1957) Genetic-statistical data on the presence of secondary oocytary twins among non-identical twins. *Acta Genet. 7*, 39–42.

Milham, S. (1966) Symmetrical conjoined twins: an analysis of the birth records of 22 sets. *J. Pediatr., 69*, 643–7.

Millis, J. (1959) The frequency of twinning in poor Chinese in the maternity hospital, Singapore. *Ann. Hum. Genet., 23*, 171–4.

Mitchell, S.C., Sellmann, A.H., Westphal, M.C. & Park, J. (1971) Etiologic correlates in a study of congenital heart disease in 56,109 births. *Am. J. Cardiol. 28*, 653–7.

Mittler, P. (1970) Biological and social aspects of language development in twins. *Dev. Med. Child. Neurol., 12*, 741–57.

Mittler, P. (1971) *The Study of Twins.* London: Penguin Books.

Mittler, P. (1976) Language development in young twins: biological, genetic and social aspects. *Acta Genet. Med. Gemellol (Roma), 25*, 359–65.

Moore, C.M., McAdams, A.J. & Sutherland, J. (1969) Intrauterine disseminated intra-vascular coagulation: a syndrome of multiple pregnancy with a dead twin fetus. *J. Pediatr., 74*, 523–8.

Morris, N., Osborn, S.B. & Wight, H.P. (1955) Effective circulation of the uterine wall in late pregnancy measured by 24NaCl. *Lancet, i*, 323–4.

Morrison, J., Kohorn, E.I. & Blackwell, R.J. (1970) Ultrasonic scanning in obstetrics: the diagnosis of multiple pregnancy. *Aust. N.Z. J. Obstet. Gynecol., 10*, 4–6.

Morton, N.E. (1955) The inheritance of human birthweight. *Ann. Hum. Genet., 20*, 125–34.

Morton, N.E. (1962) Genetics of interracial crosses in Hawaii. *Eugenics Q., 9*, 23–4.

Muller, M. (1976) The baby killer. A War on Want investigation into the promotion and sale of powdered baby milks in the Third World. 3rd ed. London: War on Want.

Muller-Holve, W., Saling, E. & Schwarz, M. (1976) The significance of the time interval in twin delivery. *J. Perinat. Med., 4*, 100–5.

Munsinger, H. (1977) The identical-twin transfusion syndrome: a source of error in estimating I.Q. resemblance and heritability. *Ann. Hum. Genet., 40*, 307–21.

Myrianthopoulos, N.C. (1970) An epidemiologic survey of twins in a large, prospectively studied population. *Am. J. Hum. Genet., 22*, 611–29.

Myrianthopoulos, N.C. (1975) Congenital malformations in twins: Epidemiologic survey. *Birth Def. Orig. Art. Ser. XI: No. 8*, 1–29. New York: National Foundation March of Dimes.

Myrianthopoulos, N.C., Churchill, J.A. & Baszynski, A.J. (1971) Respiratory distress syndrome in twins. *Acta Genet. Med. Gemellol (Roma), 20*, 199–204.

Myrianthopoulos, N.C. & Melnick, M. (1977) Malformations in monozygotic twins: a possible example of environmental influences on the developmental genetic clock. In: *Gene-Environmental Interaction in Common Diseases*, ed. E. Inouye, & H. Nichimura, pp. 206–20. Tokyo: University of Tokyo Press.

Myrianthopoulos, N.C., Nichols, P.L. & Broman, S.H. (1976) Intellectual development of twins—comparison with singletons. *Acta Genet. Med. Gemellol (Roma), 25*, 376–80.

Naeye, R.L. (1963) Human intrauterine parabiotic syndrome and its complications. *N. Engl. J. Med., 268*, 804–9.

Naeye, R.L. (1964a) Organ composition in newborn parabiotic twins with speculation regarding neonatal hypoglycaemia. *Pediatr., 34*, 415–8.

Naeye, R.L. (1964b) The fetal and neonatal development of twins. *Pediatr., 33*, 546–53.

Naeye, R.L. (1965) Organ abnormalities in a human parabiotic syndrome. *Ann. J. Pathol., 46*, 829–42.

Naeye, R.L., Benirschke, K., Hagstrom, J.W.C. & Marcus, C.C. (1966) Intrauterine growth of twins as estimated from liveborn birth weight data. *Pediatr., 37*, 409–16.

Naeye, R. & Letts, H.W. (1964) Body measurements of fetal and neonatal twins. *Arch. Pathol., 77*, 393–6.

Nance, W.E. (1981) Malformations unique to the twinning process. In: *Twin Research 3: Twin Biology and Multiple Pregnancy.* ed. W. Nance, pp. 123–33. New York: Alan R. Liss.

National Academy of Sciences (1974) *Recommended Dietary Allowance*, 8th ed. Washington DC.

Neilson, J.P. (1982) Detection of the small-for-dates twin fetus by ultrasound. Presented at the International Workshop on Twin Pregnancies, Paris.

Nelson, C.M.K. & Bunge, R.G. (1974) Semen analysis: evidence for changing parameters of male fertility potential. *Fertil. Steril., 25*, 503–7.

Newman, H.H. (1928) Asymmetry reversal or mirror imaging in identical twins. *Biol. Bull., 55*, 298–315.

Nielsen, J. (1966) Twins in sibships with Klinefelter's syndrome. *J. Med. Genet., 3*, 114–6.

Nissen, E.D. (1958) Twins: Collision, impaction, compaction and interlocking. *Obstet. Gynecol., 11*, 514–25.

Noble, E. (1980) *Having Twins: A Parent's Guide to Pregnancy, Birth and Early Childhood.* Boston: Haughton Mifflin.

Noonan, J.A. (1978) Twins, conjoined twins and cardiac defects. *Am. J. Dis. Child., 132*, 17–18.

Nora, J.J., Gilliland, J.C., Sommerville, R.J. & McNamara, D.G. (1967) Congenital heart disease in twins. *N. Engl. J. Med., 227*, 568–71.

Norman, R.J., Joubert, S.M. (1982) Amniotic fluid phospholipids in twin pregnancies. Presented at the International Workshop on Twin Pregnancies. Paris.

Nylander, P.P.S. (1967) Twinning in West Africa. *World Med. J., 14*, 178–80.

Nylander, P.P.S. (1970a) Twinning in Nigeria. *Acta Genet. Med. Gemellol (Roma), 19*, 457–64.

Nylander, P.P.S. (1970*b*) Placental forms and zygosity determination of twins in Ibadan Western Nigeria. *Acta Genet. Med. Gemellol. (Roma)*, *19*, 49–54.

Nylander, P.P.S. (1970*c*) A simple method for determining monochorionic and dichorionic placentation in twins. *Niger. J. Sci.*, *4*, 239–44.

Nylander, P.P.S. (1971*a*) The incidence of triplets and higher multiple births in some rural and urban populations in Western Nigeria. *Ann. Hum. Genet.*, *34*, 409–15.

Nylander, P.P.S. (1971*b*) Biosocial aspects of multiple births. *J. Biosoc. Sci. Suppl.*, *3*, 29–38.

Nylander, P.P.S. (1973) Serum levels of gonadotrophins in relation to multiple pregnancy in Nigeria. *J. Obstet. Gynaecol. Br. Cwlth.*, *80*, 651–3.

Nylander, P.P.S. (1975*a*) The causation of twinning. In: *Human Multiple Reproduction*, I. MacGillivray, P.P.S. Nylander & G. Corney, Chapter 4, pp. 77–86. London: W.B. Saunders.

Nylander, P.P.S. (1975*b*) Frequency of multiple births. In: *Human Multiple Reproduction*, I. MacGillivray, P.P.S. Nylander & G. Corney, Chapter 5. pp. 87–97. London: W.B. Saunders.

Nylander, P.P.S. (1975*c*) Factors which influence twinning rates. In: *Human Multiple Reproduction*, I. MacGillivray, P.P.S. Nylander & G. Corney. Chapter 6, pp. 98–106. London: W.B. Saunders.

Nylander, P.P.S. (1978) Causes of high twinning frequencies in Nigeria. *Prog. Clin. Biol. Res.*, *246*, 35–43.

Nylander, P.P.S. (1979) The twinning incidence in Nigeria. *Acta Genet. Med. Gemellol. (Roma)*, *28*, 261–3.

Nylander, P.P.S. & Corney, G. (1971) Placentation and zygosity of triplets and higher multiple births in Ibaden, Nigeria. *Ann. Hum. Genet.*, *34*, 417–27.

Nylander, P.P.S. and Corney, G. (1977) Placentation and zygosity of twins in Northern Nigeria. *Ann. Hum. Genet.*, *40*, 323–9.

Nylander, P.P.S. & MacGillivray, I. (1975*a*) The causation of twinning. In: *Human Multiple Reproduction*, MacGillivray, I., Nylander, P.P.S. & Corney, G., Chapter 4, pp. 77–86. London: W.B. Saunders.

Nylander, P.P.S. & MacGillivray, I. (1975*b*) Complications of twin pregnancy. In: *Human Multiple Reproduction*, eds. I. MacGillivray, P.P.S. Nylander & G. Corney, Chapter 10, pp. 137–46. London: W.B. Saunders.

Nylander, P.P.S. & Osunkoya, B.O. (1970) Unusual monochorionic placentation with heterosexual twins. *Obstet. Gynecol.*, *36*, 621–5.

Obladen, M. & Gluck, L. (1977) RDS and tracheal phospholipid composition in twins: independent of gestational age. *Pediatrics*, *90*, 799–802.

O'Connor, M.C., Murphy, H. & Dalrymple, I.J. (1979) Double blind trial of Ritodrine and placebo in twin pregnancy. *Br. J. Obstet. Gynaecol.*, *86*, 706–9.

Onyskowová, Z., Doležal, A. & Jedlicka, V. (1971) The frequency and the character of malformations in multiple birth (a preliminary report). *Teratology*, *4*, 496–7.

Parmar, V.T. & Mulgund, S.V. (1968) Interlocking of twin pregnancy in uterus circuatus subseptus. *J. Postgrad. Med. 14*, 139–41.

Parsons, P.A. (1965) Birth weights and survival of unlike sexed twins. *Ann. Hum. Genet.*, *28*, 1–10.

Patten, P.T. (1970) Perinatal mortality by birth order in multiple pregnancy. *Aust. N.Z. J. Obstet. Gynaecol.*, *10*, 17–9.

Penrose, L.S. (1937) Congenital syphilis in monovular twin. *Lancet*, *i*, 322.

Pepper, C.K. (1967) Ethical and moral considerations in the separation of conjoined twins. In: *Conjoined Twins*, ed. D. Bergsma. Birth Defects. Original Article Series 3: No. 1. New York: The National Foundation.

Perez, L.V., Gallo, A.D. (1965) Transfusion fetofetal. *Rev. Chile Pediatr.*, *36*, 497–500.

Phillips, C.J. (1981*a*) Mental development in the 'twin situation' a study of matched groups of twins and singletons. In: *Twins Research* (Birmingham 1968–72) Vol. 2, ed. C.J. Phillips, Part 3, pp. 189–223. Centre for Child Study University of Birmingham.

Phillips, C.J. (1981*b*) Some observations of handedness in twin children. In: *Twins Research* (Birmingham 1968–72) Vol. 2, ed. C.J. Phillips, Part V, pp. 243–72. Centre for Child Study University of Birmingham.

Phillips, C.J. & Watkinson, M. (1981) Characteristics of the families and similarity of environment within twin pairs. In: *Twins Research* (Birmingham 1968–72) Vol. 2, ed. C.J. Phillips, Part 1, pp. 2–57. Centre for Child Study University of Birmingham.

Ping, Y.W. & Chin, C.L. (1967) Incidence of twin births among the Chinese in Taiwan. *Am. J. Obstet. Gynecol.*, *98*, 881–4.

Plomin, R., Willerman, L. & Loehlin, J.C. (1976) Resemblances in appearance and the equal environments assumption in twin studies of personality traits. *Behav. Genet.*, *6*, 43–52.

Pochedly, C. & Musiker, S. (1970) Twin to twin transfusion syndrome. *Postgrad. Med.*, *47*, 172–6.

Portes, L. & Granjon, A. (1946) Les présentations au cours des accouchements gémellaires. *Gynécologie et Obstetrique*, *45*, 159–69.

Potter, E.L. (1963) Twin zygosity and placental form in relation to the outcome of pregnancy. *Am. J. Obstet. Gynecol.*, *87*, 566–77.

Potter, E.L. & Fuller, H. (1949) Multiple pregnancies at the Chicago Lying-in Hospital 1941–47. *Am. J. Obstet. Gynecol.*, *58*, 139–46.

Powell, T.J. (1981) *Symptoms of atypical depression in mothers of twins.* MSc thesis, University of Surrey.

Prokop, V.O. & Herrmann, U. (1973) Blutgruppenbefunde bei Ächtlingen. *Zentralbl. Gynäkol.*, *95*, 1497.

Quigley, J.K. (1935) Monoamniotic twin pregnancy. *Am. J. Obstet. Gynecol.*, *29*, 354–62.

Race, R.R. & Sanger, R. (1975) Blood groups in twins and chimeras. In: *Blood Groups in Man*, Chapter 26, pp. 511–46. 6th ed. Oxford: Blackwell Scientific.

Rajegowda, B.K., Freedman, M.D., Falciglia, H., Exconde, M. & Sukumaran, T. (1975) Absence of respiratory distress syndrome following premature rupture of membranes in one sib of a set of twins in two cases. *Clin. Res.*, *23*, 600A.

Ramzin, M.S., Stucki, D., Napflin, S., Allemann, F. & Gamper, S. (1982) Early prenatal loss in twin pregnancies. Presented at the International Workshop on Twin Pregnancies, Paris.

Rausen, A.R., Seki, M. & Strauss, L. (1965) Twin transfusion syndrome. A review of 19 cases studied at one institution. *J. Pediatr.*, *66*, 613–28.

Record, R.G., McKeown, T. & Edwards, J.H. (1970) An investigation of the difference in measured intelligences between twins and single birth. *Ann. Hum. Genet.*, *34*, 11–20.

Redford, D.H.A. (1982) Ultrasound assessment of uterine growth in twin pregnancy. Presented at the International Workshop on Twin Pregnancies, Paris.

Registrar General (1979) *Birth Statistics*, Series 6, p. 70. Offices of Population Census and Surveys: H.M.S.O.

Rehan, N.E., Sobrero, A.J. & Fertig, J.W. (1975) The semen of fertile men. Statistical analysis of 1,300 men. *Fertil. Steril.*, *26*, 492–502.

Reisman, L.E. & Pathak, A. (1966) Bilateral renal/cortical necrosis in the newborn. *Am. J. Dis. Child.*, *111*, 541–3.

Reisner, S.H., Forbes, A.E. & Cornblath, M. (1965) The smaller of twins and hypoglycaemia. *Lancet*, *i*, 524–6.

Reveley, A.M., Gurling, H.M.D. & Murray, R.M. (1981) Mortality and psychosis in twins. In: *Twin Research 3. Epidemiological and Clinical Studies*, ed. W. Nance, pp. 175–8. New York: Alan R. Liss.

Rhine, S.A. & Nance, W.E. (1976) Familial twinning: a case of superfetion in man. *Acta Genet. Med. Gemellol. (Roma)*, *25*, 66–9.

Riekhof, P.L., Horton, W.A., Harris, D.J. & Schimke, R.N. (1972) Monozygotic twins with the Turner Syndrome. *Am. J. Obstet. Gynecol.*, *112*, 59–61.

Rife, D.C. (1940) Handedness with special reference to twins. *Genetics*, *25*, 178–86.

Robinson, H.P. & Caines, J.S. (1977) Sonar evidence of early pregnancy failure in patients with twin conceptions. *Br. J. Obstet. Gynaecol.*, *84*, 22–5.

Robson, K.S. & Moss, H.A. (1970) Patterns and determinants of maternal attachment. *J. Pediatr.*, *77*, 976–85.

Rola-Janicki, A. (1974) Multiple births in Poland 1949–1971. In: *Multiple Births and Twin Care*, ed. P. Parisi. *Acta Genet. Med. Gemellol* (Suppl) 22

Ross, W.F. (1952) Twin pregnancy in the African. *Br. Med. J.*, *2*, 1336–7.

Rothman, K.J. (1977) Fetal loss, twinning and birth weight after oral-contraceptive use. *N. Engl. J. Med.*, *297*, 408–71.

Rowland, C. (1981) *Starting School: Together or Apart?* England: TCA leaflet.

Rudolph, A.J., Michaels, J.P. & Nichols, B.L. (1967) Obstetric management of conjoined twins. In: *Conjoined Twins*. ed. D. Bergsma. Birth Defects. Original article Series 3, No. 1. New York: The National Foundation.

Russell, E.M. (1961) Cerebral palsied twins (1961) *Arch. Dis. Child.*, *36* 328–36.

Sacks, M.O. (1959) Occurrence of anaemia and polycythemia in phenotypically dissimilar single ovum twins. *Pediatrics*, *24*, 604–8.

Salariya, E.M., Easton, P.M. & Cater, J.I. (1978) Duration of breast feeding after early initiation and frequent feeding. *Lancet*, *ii*, 1141–3.

Satge, P., Corréa, P., Charreau, M., Quénum, C. & Sanokho, A. (1966) A propos de deux cas de maladies des inclusions cytomégaliques et en particulier d'une forme subaïque encéphalique et anictérique chez un nouveau-né africain jumeau di-zygote. *Bullétin de la Société Médicale d'Afrique Noire de Lange Francaise*, *11*, 41–53.

Savić, S. (1980) *How Twins Learn to Talk*. London: Academic Press.

Scarr, S. (1969) Effects of birth weight on later intelligence. *Soc. Biol.*, *16*, 249–56.

Schatz, F. (1900) Klinische Beiträge zur Physiologie des Fötus. Berlin: A Hirschwald.

Scheinfeld, A. (1973) *Twins and Supertwins*. London: Penguin Books.

Schinzel, A.A.G.L., Smith, D.W. & Miller, J.R. (1979) Monozygotic twinning and structural defects. *J. Pediatr.*, *95*, 921–30.

Schmidt. M. & Salzano, F.M. (1980) Dissimilar effects of thalidomide in dizygotic twins. *Acta Genet. Med. Gemellol (Roma)*, *29*, 295–7.

Schneider, L. (1978) Echographic study of twin fetal growth : a plea for specific charts for twins. *Prog. Clin. Biol. Res.*, *24*, 137–41.

Schneider, L., Bessis, R. & Simmonet, T. (1979) The frequency of ovular resorption during first trimester of twin pregnancy. *Act Genet. Med. Gemmellol (Roma)*, *28*, 271–2.

Scobie, W. (1979) A language just for two. In: *Observer Magazine, May 20*, 67–9.

Scott, J.M. & Ferguson-Smith, M.A. (1973) Heterokaryotypic monozygotic twins and the acardiac monster. *J. Obstet. Gynaecol. Br. Cwlth.*, *80*, 52–9.

Scott, J.M. & Paterson, L. (1966) Monozygous anencephalic triplets—a case report. *J Obstet. Gynaecol. Br. Cwlth.*, *73*, 147–51.

Scottish Council for Research in Education (1953) Social implications of the 1947 Scottish mental survey. University of London Press.

Segreti, W.O., Winter, P.M. & Nance, W.E. (1978) Familial studies of monozygotic twinning. *Prog. Clin. Biol. Res.*, *24b.*, 55–60.

Seki, M. & Strauss, L. (1964) Absence of one umbilical artery. Analysis of 60 cases with emphasis on associated developmental aberrations. *Arch. Pathol.*, *78*, 446–53.

Shapiro, L.R., Zemek, L. & Schulman, M.J. (1978) Familial monozygotic twinning: an autosomal dominant form of monozygotic twinning with variable penetrance. *Prog. Clin Biol. Res.*, *24*, 57–62.

Shearer, W.T., Schreiner, R.I., Marshall, R.E. & Barton, L.L. (1972) Cytomegalovirus infection in a newborn dizygotic twin. *J: Pediatr.*, *81*, 1161–5.

Shorland, J. (1971) Management of the twin transfusion syndrome. *Clin. Pediatr.*, *10*, 160–3

Sims, C.D., Cowan, D.B. & Parkinson, C.E. (1976) The lecithin/sphingomyelin ratio in twin pregnancies. *Br. J. Obstet. Gynaecol.*, *83*, 447–51.

Sinha, D.P., Nandakumar, V.C. & Beebeejaun, M.S. (1979) Relative cervical incompetence in twin pregnancy. *Acta Genet. Med. Gemellol. (Roma).*, *28*, 327–31.

Sinykin, M.B. (1958) Monoamniotic triplet pregnancy with triple survival. *Obstet. Gynecol.*, *12*, 78–82.

Skerlj, B. (1939) Menarche und Umvelt. *Z. Menschl Vererb-Konstit Lehre*, *23*, 299–359.

Smellie, W.A. (1752) *A Treatise on the Theory and Practice of Midwifery*, 2nd ed. London : Wilson and Durham.

Smith, A. (1966) Observations on the determinants of human multiple births. In: *Annual Report of the Registrar General for Scotland 1964*.

Smith, D.W., Bartlett, C. & Harrah, L.M. (1976) Monozygotic twinning and the Duhamel anomalad (imperforate anus to sirenomelia) A non-random association between two aberrations in morphogenesis. *Birth Defects, 12*, 53–63.

Smith, S.M. & Penrose, L.S. (1955) Monozygotic and dizygotic twin diagnosis. *Ann. Hum. Genet., 19*, 273–89.

Social Services Committee Report on Perinatal and Neonatal Mortality (1980) Vol. 1, para. 326, p. 101. HMSO.

Soma, H., Takayama, M., Kiyokawa, T., Akaeda, T. & Tokoro, K. (1975) Serum gonadotropin levels in Japanese women. *Obstet. Gynecol., 46*, 311–2.

Sorgo, G. (1973) Das Problem der Superfoecundatio in Vaterschaftsgutachten. *Beitr. Gerichtl. Med., 30*, 415–21.

Spellacy, W.N., Cruz, A.C., Buhi, W.C. & Birk, S.A. (1977) Amniotic fluid L/S ratio in twin gestation. *Obstet. Gynecol., 50*, 68.

Spiers, P.S. (1974) Estimated rates of concordancy for the sudden infant death syndrome in twins. *Am. J. Epidemiol., 100*, 1–7.

Spurway, J.H. (1962) The fate and management of the second twin. *Am. J. Obstet. Gynecol., 83*, 1377–88.

Stables, J. (1980) Breastfeeding Twins. In: *Nursing Times*, 1493–4.

Statistical Bulletin of the Metropolitan Life Insurance Co. (1960).

Stevenson, A.C., Johnston, H.A., Stewart, M.I.P. & Golding, D.R. (1966) Congenital malformations. A report of a study of series of consecutive births in 24 centres. *Bull. Wld. Hlth. Org., 34*, Suppl.

Stevenson, J. (1982) Study of 13 year old twins and their reading development. Hospital for Sick Children, Great Ormond Street, London.

Stockard, C.R. (1921) Developmental rate and structural expression: an experimental study of twins, 'double monsters' and single deformities, and the interaction among embryonic organs during their origin and development. *Am. J. Anat., 28*, 115–277.

Strong, S.J. & Corney, G. (1967) *The Placenta in Twin Pregnancy*. Oxford: Pergamon Press.

Stucki, D., Ramzin, M.S. & Zehnder, A. (1982) Management of twin pregnancies. Presented at the International Workshop on Twin Pregnancies, Paris.

Tagawa, T. (1974) Monoamniotic twins with a double survival. Report of a case with a peculiar cord complication. *Wis. Med. J., 73*, 131–2.

Tan, K-L., Tan, R., Tan, S.H. & Tan, A.M. (1979) The twin transfusion syndrome. *Clin. Pediatr., 18*, 111–4.

Tan, K-L., Tock, E.P.C., Dawood, M.Y. & Ratnam, S. (1971) Conjoined twins in a triplet pregnancy. *Am. J. Dis. Child., 122*, 455–8.

Tanner, J.M. Healy, M.J.R., Lockhart, R.D., MacKenzie, J.D. & Whitehouse, R.H. (1956) The prediction of adult body measurements taken each year from birth to 5 years. *Arch. Dis. Child., 31*, 372–81.

Terasaki, P.I., Gjertson, D., Bernoco, D., Perdue, S., Mickey, M.R. & Bond, J. (1978) Twins with two different fathers identified by HLA. *N. Engl. J. Med., 299*, 590–2.

Theron, J.P. (1969) A case of locked twins in a double uterus. *J. Obstet. Gynaecol., Br. Cwlth., 76*, 750–1.

Thomsen, R.J. (1978) Delayed interval delivery of a twin pregnancy. *Obstet. Gynecol., 52 (suppl.)*, 375–405.

Timonen, S. & Carpen, E. (1968) Multiple pregnancies and photoperiodicity. *Ann. Chir. Gynaec. Fenn., 57*, 135–8.

Topping, C. (1982) Guide for mothers of supertwins. England: Twins Clubs Association.

Torgersen, J. (1950) Situs inversus, asymmetry, and twinning. *Am. J. Hum. Genet., 2*, 361–70.

Tow, S.H. (1959) Fetal wastage in twin pregnancy. *J. Obstet. Gynaecol., J. Br. Emp., 66*, 444–51.

Turksoy, R.N., Toy, B.L., Rogers, J. & Papageorge, W. (1967) Birth of septuplets following gonadotrophin administration in Chiari–Frommel syndrome. *Obstet. Gynecol., 30*, 692–8.

Twins Clubs Association (1981) Hints and advice on bottle feeding twins. England: TCA leaflet.

Tyson, J.E. (1976) In Breastfeeding and the Mother. Ciba Foundation Symposium 45 (new ser.). London: Elsevier.

Valaes, T. & Doxiadis, S.A., (1960) Intrauterine blood transfer between uniovular twins *Arch. Dis. Child.*, *35*, 503–5.

Vandenberg, S.G. & Falkner, F. (1966) Hereditary factors in human growth. *Hum. Biol.*, *37*, 357–65.

Vestergaard, P. (1972) Triplets pregnancy with a normal foetus and a dicephalus dibrachius sirenomelus. *Acta Obstet. Gynecol. Scand.*, *51*, 93–4.

Wald, N.J., Cuckle, H., Stirrat, G.M., Bennett, M.J. & Turnbull, A.C. (1977) Maternal serum alphafetoprotein and low birthweight. *Lancet*, *ii*, 268–70.

Wald, N.J., Cuckle, H., Stirrat, G.M. & Turnbull, A.C. (1978) Maternal serum alphafetoprotein and birthweight in twin pregnancies. *Br. J. Obstet. Gynaecol.*, *85*, 582–4.

Wald, N.J., Cuckle, H.S. Peck, S., Stirrat, G.M. & Turnbull, A.C. (1979) Maternal serum alphafetoprotein in relation to zygosity. *Br. Med. J.*, *1*, 455.

Walker, J., & Turnbull, C.P. (1955) The environment of the foetus in human multiple pregnancy. *Etudes Néonatales*, *4*, 123–48.

Weekes, A.R.L., Cheridjian, V.E. & Mwanje, D.K. (1977a) Lumbar epidural analgesia in labour in twin pregnancy. *Br. Med. J.*, *2*, 730–2.

Weekes, A.R.L., Menzies, D.N., & de Boer, C.H. (1977b) The relative efficacy of bed rest, cervical suture and no treatment in the management of twin pregnancy. *Br. J. Obstet Gynaecol.*, *84*, 161–4.

Weekes, A.R.L., Menzies, D.N. & West, C.R. (1977c) Spontaneous premature birth in twin pregnancy. *Br. Med. J.* *2*, 14–17.

Weinberg, W. (1902) Beiträge zur Physiologie und Pathologie der Mehrlingsgeburten beim Menschen. *Pflügers Archiv fur die gesamte physiologie de Menschen und der Tiere*, *88*, 346–430.

Weir, P.E., Ratten, G.J. & Beischer, N.A. (1979) Acute polyhydramios—a complication of monozygous twin pregnancy. *Br. J. Obstet. Gynaecol.*, *86*, 849–53.

Welch, P., Black, K.N. & Christian, J.C. (1978) Placental type and Bayley Mental Development scores in 18-month-old twins. *Prog. Clin. Biol. Res.*, *24*, 145–9.

Weller, P.H., Jenkins, P.A., Gupta, J. & Baum, J.D. (1976) Pharyngeal lecithin sphing-omyelin ratios in newborn infants. *Lancet*, *i*, 12–5.

Wharton, B., Edwards, J.H. & Cameron, A.H. (1968) Monoamniotic twins. *J. Obstet. Gynecol*, *75*, 158–63.

White, C. and Wyshak, G. (1964) Inheritance of human dizygotic twinning. *N. Engl. J. Med.*, *271*, 1003–5.

Whitehouse, D.B.B. & Kohler, H.G. (1960) Vasa praevia in twin pregnancy: report of two cases. *J. Obstet. Gynecol, Br. Emp.*, *67*, 281–3.

Willerman, L. & Churchill, J.A. (1967) Intelligence and birth weight in identical twins. *Child. Devel.*, *38*, 623–9.

Williams, B. & Cummings, G. (1953) Unusual case of twins: case report. *J. Obstet. Gynaecol. Br. Emp.*, 60, 319–21.

Wilson, R.S. (1974a) Growth standards for twins from birth to four years. *Ann. Hum. Biol.*, *1* 175–88.

Wilson, R.S. (1974b) Twins: mental development in the pre-school years. *Devel. Psychol.*, *10*, 580–8.

Wilson, R.S. (1978) Synchronies in mental development. An epigenetic perspective. *Science*, *202*, 939–47.

Wilson, R.S. (1979) Twin growth: initial deficit, recovery and trends in concordance from birth to nine years. *Ann. Hum. Biol.*, *6*, 205–20.

Wilson, R.S. (1981) Synchronised developmental pathways for infant twins. In: *Twin Research 3. Intelligence, Personality and Development.* ed. W. Nance, pp. 199–209. New York: Alan R. Liss.

Wilson, R.S., Brown, A.M. & Matheny, A.P. (1971) Emergence and persistence of behavioural differences in twins. *J. Child. Devel.* *42*, 1381–98.

Wolkind, S. (1981) Depression in mothers of young children. *Arch. Dis. Child.*, *56*, 1–3.

Woods, D.L. & Malan, A.F. (1977) Assessment of gestational age in twins. *Arch. Dis. Child.*, *52*, 735–7.

Woods, D.L. & Malan, A.F. (1980) Superfecundation. *Arch. Dis. Child.*, *55*, 974.

Wyshak, G. (1978) Menopause in mothers of multiple births and mothers of singletons only. *Soc. Biol.*, *25*, 52–61.

Wyshak, G. (1981) Reproductive and menstrual characteristics of mothers of multiple births and mothers of singletons only: a discriminant analysis. In: *Twin Research 3. Twin Biology and Multiple Pregnancy*, ed. W. Nance, pp. 95–105. New York: Alan R. Liss.

Wyshak, G. and White, C. (1963) Birth hazard of the second twin. *J. Am. Med. Assoc.*, *186*, 869–70.

Wyshak, G. & White, C. (1965a) Number of sibs preceding, and number following, the birth of twins. *Ann. Hum. Genet.*, *28*, 357–9.

Wyshak, G. & White, C. (1965b) Genealogical study of human twinning. *Am. J. Public Health*, *55*, 1586–93.

Yoshioka, H., Kadomoto, Y., Mino, M., Morikawa, Y., Kasubuchi, Y. & Kusonoki, T. (1979) Multicystic encephalomalacia in liveborn twin with a stillborn macerated co-twin. *J. Pediatr.*, *95*, 798–800.

Yue, S.J. (1955) Multiple births in cerebral palsy. *Am. J. Phys. Med.*, *34*, 335–41.

Zazzo, R., (1960) Les Jumeaux: Le Couple et la Personne. Paris: Presse Universitaire de France.

Zazzo, R. (1979) The twin condition and the couple effect on personality development. *Acta Genet. Med. Gemellol. (Roma)*, *25*, 343–52.

Zuckerman, H. & Brzezinski, A. (1961) Multiple Pregnancies. *Isr. Med. J.*, *20*, 251–8.

Index

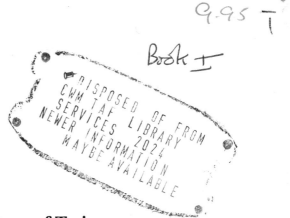
The Nature and Nurture of Twins

To Pamela Davies